Snoring and Sleep Apnea

Personal and Family Guide
to Diagnosis and Treatment

Ralph A. Pascualy, M.D.
Sally Warren Soest, M.S.

Foreword by William C. Dement, M.D., Ph.D.

demos vermande

Demos Vermande, 386 Park Avenue South, New York, New York 10016

Made in the United States of America.

Illustrations: Robert Holmberg, University of Washington,
Health Sciences Center for Educational Resources

Photographs: 6.1, 6.2, 6.3, 6.4, 6.5, 6.6 by Gayle Rieber Photography
                 7.1 (A) from video by Dr. Stephen B. Anderson
                 7.2 Photographs courtesy of:
                     (A) ResCare, Ltd.
                     (B) Lifecare
                     (C) Respironics, Inc.
                     (D) Healthdyne Technologies
                     (E) Puritan-Bennett
                 7.3 Photographs courtesy of:
                     (A) Puritan-Bennett
                     (B) ResCare, Ltd.
                     (C) Lifecare
                     (D) Healthdyne Technologies
                     (E) Respironics, Inc.
                 7.6 (A, B) courtesy of Dr. Nelson Powell
                 9.1, 9.2, 14.1 courtesy of ResCare, Ltd.

Video capture: 7.1 (A, B) Joseph Wilmhoff, University of Washington,
               Health Sciences Center for Educational Resources.

Library of Congress Cataloging in Publication Data
Pascualy, Ralph A., 1951-
         Snoring and sleep apnea : personal and family guide to diagnosis
     and treatment / Ralph A. Pascualy, Sally Warren Soest ; foreword by
     William C. Dement. — 2nd ed.
         p.   cm
     Includes bibliographical references and index.
     ISBN 0-939957-82-5 (softcover)
         1. sleep apnea syndromes — Popular works. 2. Snoring — Popular
     works.   I. Soest, Sally Warren, 1942-   . II. Title.
     RC737.5.P37   1996
     616.8' 498—dc20   95-46517
                                                  CIP

Contents

Foreword

Sleep apnea syndrome is number one among the hundred-plus sleep disorders recognized today. Why?

1. Sleep apnea is common: it affects one in ten middle-aged men. It is slightly less common in women.
2. Sleep apnea, untreated, can be deadly.
3. Sleep apnea patients are poorly diagnosed and treated because of the lack of trained sleep experts.

Sleep apnea robs people of vitality, health, and sometimes life itself. Loss of vitality will be familiar to many readers of this book. People suffering from sleep apnea fall asleep anywhere and everywhere, even while driving. Their heavy snoring disrupts their own sleep and often that of their family. They drag themselves to work despite exhaustion, doze at their desks, stumble home completely drained, and fall asleep on the sofa. They lack the energy to enjoy family life or the company of friends.

The health consequences of sleep apnea are even more grave. Untreated sleep apnea puts people at high risk for driving accidents, high blood pressure, stroke, irregular heart rhythms, and other life-threatening complications.

Treatment is available and dramatically effective. Formerly sick, sleepy people quickly regain their vigor, resume their cherished activities, and thrive. Life is restored.

Accurate diagnosis is the major problem. Eighty to ninety percent of sleep apnea victims are still undiagnosed. The National Commission on Sleep Disorders Research heard countless witnesses testify to suffering for ten years or more before sleep apnea was correctly diagnosed and treated.

My primary mission in life today is to lift the shroud of darkness surrounding sleep disorders, and with it years of prolonged and needless suffering. Education is the key: public education, patient education, and medical education.

This book answers all three of those educational needs. It educates the sleep apnea sufferer and the public alike. Further, the book is an authoritative survey of sleep apnea diagnosis and treatment for the primary care physician.

Ralph Pascualy and Sally Soest have produced a much needed guide for people who suspect they have sleep apnea, for people who have been diagnosed, and for those undertaking lifelong treatment.

I can recommend this book to all those with sleep apnea and their friends and families. Use it as a pathfinder. Let it point the way out of the twilight of sleep apnea to timely diagnosis, appropriate treatment, and a bright future.

William C. Dement, M.D., Ph.D.
Chairman, National Commission on Sleep Disorders Research
Palo Alto, California

Preface

The Inspiration

This book was born in the convergence of two separate viewpoints: doctor and patient. One of the authors (SWS) is married to a person who has sleep apnea. The other author (RAP) is the sleep disorders specialist who diagnosed and treated him. The two authors met across an information gap. They wrote this book in a combined effort to bridge that gap.

The need for this book was clear to Sally Soest from the day her husband heard, by chance, about sleep apnea: a newspaper story told of a truck driver who kept falling asleep at the wheel. Seeking additional information, the author discovered that little was written about sleep apnea except in specialized sleep medicine journals. Sleep apnea was surrounded by an information vacuum: scant public awareness, no guideposts for the patient, and poor recognition even in the medical community.

The author learned that this absence of information has a price. A surprising twenty million Americans have this potentially fatal disorder, yet ninety percent are still undiagnosed. Some of those unsuspecting people will die prematurely from the effects of unrecognized, untreated sleep apnea: a high price to pay for lack of information.

As the author met other sleep apnea patients, she became aware of a typical pattern. The most common means of diagnosis seemed to be self-diagnosis by chance, by the patient himself or by a loved one. However, prior to that many people have spent years seeking the correct diagnosis while doctors treated the symptoms, without associating them with sleep apnea. For his heavy snoring, a patient might be advised to try a decongestant, or to tell his wife to sleep in the guest room. For his weight problems, he might be told, "Lose weight." For his heart problems, he might receive a prescription for heart medication; for his drowsiness, a stimulant; for his sleep complaints, a sleeping pill. Meanwhile, the patient felt worse and the untreated sleep apnea progressed.

Once a person has received a diagnosis of sleep apnea, the absence of reliable patient support literature has left him without the means to understand this complex disorder, to choose the appropriate treatment, and to deal with long-term issues.

As a sleep disorders specialist, Ralph Pascualy has struggled continually to fill the sleep apnea information vacuum, trying both to provide meaningful patient education material and to raise the level of awareness within the medical community.

The two authors agreed that it was time for a clear, authoritative book written for people with actual or suspected sleep apnea, for their spouses, and for family doctors alike, to help them understand sleep apnea and lead them toward more timely diagnosis and appropriate, successful treatment.

The Message

❖   Sleep apnea is:
        surprisingly common,
        debilitating,
        potentially fatal,
        treatable,
        frequently unrecognized by family doctors.

❖   If you have the symptoms described in Chapter 1, act now. Take the initiative, schedule a sleep test, and find out if you have sleep apnea.

❖   Don't waste your prime years. Treatment of sleep apnea can restore health and vigor, so you have the energy to do the things you enjoy in life.

❖   Have your sleep test done by a qualified sleep specialist.

What This Book Will Do for You

The following chapters describe the causes and consequences of sleep apnea, the tests for diagnosing sleep apnea, and pro's and con's of current treatments.

Chapter 12 tells how to find a qualified sleep specialist and the nearest accredited sleep testing center.

Chapters 13 through 15 contain suggestions about living with sleep apnea and dealing with the treatment process, plus information on products and services for people who are being treated for sleep apnea.

The names of patients have been changed to preserve their privacy. Also, in the interest of simplicity and because sleep apnea is more common among males, patients usually have been referred to as "he" and their partners as "she." This should not be interpreted to imply any disregard for the many women who have sleep apnea and their caring, supportive male partners.

You can free yourself from the twilight world of lifeless days and tortured nights. Make an appointment at the nearest accredited sleep center. Do it now.

Ralph A. Pascualy, M.D.
Seattle, WA

Sally Warren Soest
Seattle, WA

➤ ➤ ➤ ➤ ➤ 1 ➤ ➤ ➤ ➤ ➤

Do You Have Sleep Apnea?

WHAT IS SLEEP APNEA?

Sleep apnea (pronounced "AP-nee-uh") is a breathing disorder that affects people while they sleep, usually without their knowing it. The most common symptom is loud, heavy snoring, which is often treated as a joke. But sleep apnea is no joking matter, for it can often result in heart problems, automobile accidents, strokes, and death. Sleep apnea is a potentially fatal disorder.

People with sleep apnea stop breathing repeatedly during a night's sleep. [The word *apnea* comes from the Greek prefix *a* ("no") and the Greek word *pnoia* ("breath").] Breathing may stop ten, 20, or even 100 or more times per hour of sleep and may not start again for a minute or longer. As you can imagine, these sleep/breathing disruptions deprive the person of both sleep and oxygen.

This may not sound terribly serious. "So what?" you may think. "So the person is a little tired or sleepy during the day. What's the problem?"

The problem is twofold. First, sleep apnea is a serious health hazard. Second, a stunning number of people have sleep apnea and don't know it: between 20 million and 25 million Americans. In a recent study of 30- to 60-year-olds, 24% of the men and 9% of the women had signs of sleep apnea.[1]

1

A disturbing study of a group of truckers showed that 87% had signs of sleep apnea.[2] This is a tragedy in the making, because people with untreated sleep apnea are at high risk of falling asleep at the wheel, and when a trucker dies behind the wheel he sends an average of 4.3 innocent victims to their graves.

Unless it is properly treated, sleep apnea can cause:

✦ Irregular heartbeat.

✦ High blood pressure.

✦ Enlargement of the heart.

✦ Increased risk of heart failure.

✦ Increased risk of stroke.

✦ Excessive sleepiness.

✦ Workplace and automobile accidents.

✦ Impotence.

✦ Uncontrollable weight gain.

✦ Psychological symptoms, such as irritability and
   depression.

✦ Deterioration of memory, alertness, and coordination.

✦ Death.

Untreated sleep apnea can be progressive, worsening over the course of ten or 20 years, until it presents a real threat to life.

> **Case Study.** *On the Wednesday before Christmas of 1985, Reverend Allen felt himself slipping toward death. This 67-year-old retired minister had seen one doctor after another, searching for the reason for his declining health. Specialists had treated him for heart problems and a variety of other symptoms. But no one had been able to explain what was*

causing his problems. By December, 1985, Mr. Allen was so weak he could hardly walk across his living room.

Now his only prayer was that he might make it through Christmas.

All his life Mr. Allen had lacked energy; even a little exertion wore him out. He slept poorly and never awakened refreshed. When he had retired from preaching, he had looked forward to getting plenty of rest and finally feeling better. Instead he had felt more exhausted than ever. His health had grown much worse.

He began to lose his coordination. Simple things, such as walking and writing, became difficult. His memory was failing and he would forget familiar words. This embarrassed and saddened him, for he had been a skilled craftsman with words, a preacher's most powerful tools. But now those tools seemed scattered and lost. Even his sense of humor had disappeared.

The previous summer his wife had noticed a story in an insurance company magazine about a disorder called sleep apnea. The symptoms had rung a familiar bell: heavy snoring, daytime sleepiness, and exhaustion. She had awakened Mr. Allen, who was asleep as usual in his easy chair, and suggested that he might find the article interesting.

Indeed he did! The article described him exactly. Excited and hopeful, Mr. Allen took the article to his doctor. But his doctor was not particularly interested.

The next six months became a race with time, as Mr. Allen's health rapidly deteriorated. His wife doggedly pursued their only lead, sleep apnea, through a long string of discouraging phone calls. Finally, they were put in touch with a new sleep disorders center in a nearby city. They made an appointment for an interview on the Wednesday before Christmas.

On the appointment day Mr. Allen seemed so frail that his wife was afraid he might die on the way to the sleep center. She nearly canceled the appointment. But Mr. Allen was determined to try to make it through Christmas. "What's the difference," he had shrugged, "whether you go to Heaven from home or from the freeway?"

The sleep specialist immediately suspected severe sleep apnea. He rearranged his schedule so that Mr. Allen could have a sleep test the very next night. The doctor knew that if he delayed, he would be sorry for a very long time.

Sleep tests revealed that Mr. Allen had severe obstructive sleep apnea. He was immediately started on treatment with CPAP, a breathing device that is used at night (see Chapter 7).

"And that," says Mr. Allen, "was a new beginning! The first morning after I went on CPAP, I woke up feeling refreshed. I wanted to take a walk!"

Three months later, this man who had been near death, barely able to shuffle across his living room, was walking three-quarters of a mile every day. And to his friends' delight and his own, his sense of humor had returned.

Reverend Allen's heart problems probably were the result of a lifetime of untreated sleep apnea. If sleep apnea is treated correctly, these medical problems can be prevented, and even reversed. The sooner treatment is begun, the better the results.

Mr. Allen's story is dramatic. Not every case of long-term sleep apnea is so severe, and not every recovery is so striking. But in many ways Mr. Allen's story is typical: the snoring, the sleepiness, the fatigue, the loss of vigor, the threatening progress of an unidentified disease, the frustrations of seeking help where none seems available.

Most sleep apnea sufferers have followed, and still follow, a similar path. We must hope that, as the public and the medical community become more aware of the signs, symptoms, and seriousness of sleep apnea, people will be diagnosed at an earlier stage and can begin treatment before they develop severe medical complications.

WHAT ARE THE SYMPTOMS OF SLEEP APNEA?

If you have sleep apnea, you may be the last person to recognize the symptoms. After all, you are asleep when many of them occur. Often it is a friend or loved one who notices that someone's sleep, or his breathing during sleep, is not quite normal.

So, husbands, wives, children, and friends: See if the ten most common symptoms of sleep apnea are familiar to you.

The first two symptoms go together.

Symptoms 1 and 2

> **Loud, irregular snoring and snorts, gasps, and other unusual breathing sounds during sleep.**

The most obvious sign of sleep apnea is very noisy snoring that stops and starts in an unrhythmic manner during the night. The snoring stops when the person stops breathing. It begins again, sometimes with a snort or a gasp, when the person takes the next breath.

Irregular snoring, with breathing that stops, is different from the quiet, relaxed sawing of ZZZ's that most of us do occasionally, especially if we're sleeping on our back. Apnea-type snoring is noisy, labored, and sometimes explosive, and strongly suggest some struggle or discomfort on the part of the snorer.

Another characteristic of severe apnea-type snoring is that the snorer seems to snore in nearly any position. Rolling over on the side often does not help, as it usually does in the case of simple, harmless nonapnea snoring. Some patients, however, snore and have apnea only when sleeping on their back.

Symptom 3

> **Pauses in breathing during sleep.**

Everyone's breathing is irregular at certain times during sleep. For example, just as you fall asleep, or as you awaken, your breathing may pause for a moment. And during periods of dreaming, your breathing tends to speed up and slow down in an irregular manner. These are all normal changes in breathing while asleep.

However, a person with sleep apnea frequently stops breathing entirely and may hold his breath for a surprisingly long time.

Each of these periods during which breathing has stopped is called an *apnea episode,* or *apnea event.* An apnea event may last from ten seconds to more than a minute.

Sleep specialists measure sleep apnea in several ways. One way is to count the number of apnea events during the night and measure how long they last. A person is considered to have signs of sleep apnea if he stops breathing for more than ten seconds at a time and if this happens more than five times during an hour of sleep. This would be a very mild case of sleep apnea, but one that would bear watching, to ensure that it did not become worse.

Apnea events do not happen just once or twice, but five, ten, 20, or more times *per hour.* In some people, apnea may occur only during part of the night; in others it can continue all night. By morning a person with sleep apnea may have experienced hundreds of fairly long periods of nonbreathing.

You might think that a person would be aware of such a struggle to breathe during sleep. Some apnea patients do notice that they awaken briefly with a snort, particularly during naps or when they nod off in a sitting position. A few people with sleep apnea will wake up completely to breathe, but usually they don't know why they have awakened. These people are likely to describe their problem as "insomnia."

However, most people with sleep apnea are *unaware of having a sleep/breathing problem.* Many have absolutely *no complaints* about their sleep. They believe they sleep "just fine," and only wish their bedpartner would stop bothering them about their snoring.

A tape recording of a person's sleeping sounds can be useful for convincing both that person and his doctor that he suffers from a breathing disorder during sleep.

Symptoms 4 and 5

(**Excessive daytime sleepiness** and/or **fatigue.**)

The most common sleep complaint of people with sleep apnea is that they get "too much sleep." Sleep specialists call this symptom *excessive daytime sleepiness (EDS).*

Two-thirds of sleep apnea patients suffer from some degree of EDS, and they may not even know it. Often people have simply lived with the effects of sleep apnea for so long, or it has crept up on them so gradually, that they do not know what "normal" feels like. They may think that they feel normal, or that drowsiness is just a sign of getting older, or that maybe they just need a vacation.

However, it is *not normal* to have to fight to stay awake at your desk at work, at the wheel while driving, at the dinner table, at parties, at sporting events. If you are struggling against sleepiness during the day, you need to find out what is causing your abnormal drowsiness. Find out now, before it further undermines your life.

EDS results mainly from poor sleep; in sleep apnea, the person's sleep is interrupted throughout the night by repeated apnea events. He doesn't get enough sleep, and his sleep is of poor quality. As a result of these sleep/breathing disturbances, someone with sleep apnea builds up a "sleep debt": an ongoing need for sleep that carries over into his daytime life. His sleep debt pressures him to fall asleep easily and frequently during the daytime: at his desk at work, while reading or watching TV, while driving.

Fatigue is another common problem for people with sleep apnea. Fatigue is different from sleepiness. Rather than a desire to go to sleep, fatigue is a sense of feeling exhausted, drained. People with sleep apnea typically feel fatigued a lot of the time. Often, because their apnea has been present for years and has gotten progressively worse, they are not even aware that they *are* more tired than normal. Or they assume that their fatigue is simply a normal sign of age.

Again, as with drowsiness, a constant feeling of exhaustion is *not normal*. It is *not* an inevitable sign of age. A person who feels fatigued a lot of the time probably has a medical problem. It may or may not be sleep apnea. But a physician should certainly consider sleep apnea as a possible cause of unexplained fatigue and refer a chronically fatigued patient to a sleep clinic for testing if he has suspicious symptoms.

Case Study. *Mr. Bell's wife pleaded with him to see a doctor about his gasping and irregular breathing during sleep. But Mr. Bell was in excellent physical condition and at the age of 46 could outrun much younger men in 10k races. He had seen a TV show about sleep problems and knew that some apnea and snoring can be normal, so he ignored his wife's request.*

A life insurance company reviewed Mr. Bell's medical records and noticed that the doctor's note suggested "possible sleep apnea," so they denied his insurance. Mr. Bell went to a sleep center, hoping to prove he was in perfect health. Instead he learned that, in fact, he had moderately severe apnea.

Mr. Bell received treatment for his sleep apnea, and a follow-up study of his sleep showed an excellent response. His insurance was approved, which pleased him; in addition, Mr. Bell realized that he felt much better. He was amazed that he had not noticed the signs of sleep apnea prior to treatment.

The moral of Mr. Bell's story is clear: if your bedpartner is concerned that you have sleep apnea, he or she may be right, even if you don't feel ill. Some people can tolerate very significant amounts of sleep apnea without being aware of it. Apparently, they do not notice a deterioration in the quality of their sleep or their daytime alertness, nor are they bothered by "insomnia" or fatigue. Mr. Bell is typical of former sleep apnea patients after treatment: they are astonished at feeling so much more wide awake, energetic, and alive.

Symptom 6

(**Obesity.**)

Obesity is fairly common among people with sleep apnea. A complicated relationship exists between weight and sleep apnea: sleep apnea makes the weight problem worse, and vice versa.

Losing weight usually helps the sleep apnea, but often people cannot lose weight until after the sleep apnea has been treated. The sleep apnea–obesity relationship is described in more detail in Chapter 8.

Not everyone who is overweight suffers from sleep apnea, nor is everyone who has sleep apnea necessarily overweight. In fact, individuals who are quite thin can have severe sleep apnea.

Case Study. Mr. Johnson was a 29-year-old who snored badly and had been tired "for years." His wife had noticed pauses in his breathing during sleep, but these were infrequent, and she was a good sleeper, so she didn't mind his snoring.

Several doctors over several years had performed thorough medical examinations and had concluded that stress or underlying depression were the likely causes of Mr. Johnson's chronic tiredness. During his last evaluation he mentioned the snoring and the apnea that his wife had observed, but he was told he was "too young and too thin" to have any trouble with sleep apnea.

Eventually, Mr. Johnson was studied in a sleep center, and it was discovered that he stopped breathing 43 times an hour. With treatment using nasal CPAP (see Chapter 7), Mr. Johnson's fatigue disappeared entirely.

Symptom 7

Changes in alertness, memory, personality, or behavior.

Sleep apnea can mimic depression, laziness, or personality change.

As with the other symptoms of sleep apnea, family and friends often are the first to notice behavioral signs of sleep apnea. These changes in behavior can include a gradual shift in sleeping or napping habits, in the person's energy level, in his productivity at home or at work, or in his mood or disposition. Any of these changes in behavior, which the person himself might not notice, may suggest sleep apnea.

Case Study. Mr. Arnold was under a lot of stress. His business was in trouble from new competition. His wife was drinking heavily, and their marriage seemed to be breaking down. His business partner was concerned that he was gaining weight, seemed irritable and depressed, and was not his usual outgoing self with the office staff and customers. In business meetings Mr. Arnold was distractible and his once photographic memory for business statistics was slipping badly.

His partner suggested that he see a psychologist and get help to deal with his stress, depression, and marital problems. He took his partner's advice. But counseling did not help, and his family doctor referred him to a psychiatrist. The psychiatrist noted his snoring and sleepiness and sent him to a sleep center for testing, where he was found to be suffering from sleep apnea. Treatment resolved his personality change, memory problems, and poor work performance.

Unexplained changes in mental sharpness or in personality should arouse a suspicion of possible sleep apnea, particularly if these changes are accompanied by apnea during sleep, fatigue, weight gain, or other symptoms mentioned in this chapter.

Increased irritability, shortness of temper, or "crabbiness" are very often caused by sleep apnea but may be explained away as the result of stress in the person's life.

Other Symptoms of Sleep Apnea (Symptoms 8, 9, and 10)

Other symptoms sometimes associated with sleep apnea are the following:

Impotence.

Morning headaches.

Bedwetting.

Few people will have all the symptoms of sleep apnea. Most people will show only one or two obvious signs of the disorder.

It is important to emphasize that any of the symptoms of sleep apnea might also be caused by other, possibly harmful conditions. For this and other reasons, a person suspected of having sleep apnea should be tested by a physician who specializes in sleep disorders, so that other disorders can be ruled out and the correct diagnosis made.

Summary

A person shows signs of sleep apnea syndrome that may affect his health:

✤ If he stops breathing for more than ten seconds at a time, and

✤ If this happens more than five times during an hour of sleep.

The following are the most common signs and symptoms of sleep apnea:

1. Loud, irregular snoring.

2. Snorts, gasps, and other unusual breathing sounds during sleep.

3. Long pauses in breathing during sleep.

4. Excessive daytime sleepiness.

5. Fatigue.

6. Obesity.

7. Changes in alertness, memory, personality, or behavior.

8. Impotence.

9. Morning headaches.

10. Bedwetting.

If you have loud, irregular snoring plus any of the other preceding symptoms, you should ask your doctor to refer you to an accredited sleep center for evaluation.

➤ ➤ ➤ ➤ ➤   2   ➤ ➤ ➤ ➤ ➤

Sleep Apnea Harms Health and Home Life

Over the years sleep apnea exacts a high price. People with it suffer significant damage from the poor quality of their sleep, from their nightly struggle to breathe, and from the lower than normal oxygen supply in their blood during the night.

The long-term damage from sleep apnea can be divided into **health effects** and **social and psychological effects**. The seriousness of the damage depends upon how long the apnea has been present and the person's overall health.

HEALTH EFFECTS OF SLEEP APNEA

Most of the serious health problems from sleep apnea develop gradually, over the long term. But one source of injury is very abrupt: the auto wreck.

Automobile Accidents

Auto accidents are extremely common among people with untreated sleep apnea. Nearly 20% of sleep apnea patients admit to having had auto accidents from falling asleep at the wheel.[1] Recent studies of long-haul truck drivers have found that 46% of the drivers had obvious symptoms of sleep apnea and that the most common single cause of heavy truck accidents was "fatigue."[2]

Sleepiness while driving usually develops gradually over weeks or months. The driver may ignore or not admit the warning signal of a potentially life-threatening episode of sleepiness.

Prior to having an actual auto accident, most if not all apnea patients have had very brief "micro-sleeps" while driving. They nod off for an instant, perhaps also experiencing a prolonged eye blink or an actual bobbing of the head. This brief sleep may result in the car wandering in the lane, drifting onto the shoulder, or even crossing into the next lane.

The family of a person with life-threatening sleepiness may have observed him repeatedly falling asleep, even on short trips; yet the driver may absolutely deny that he is sleepy or dangerous. The reasons for denial can be complicated, ranging from lack of awareness to pride to unconscious denial of the problem.

Auto accidents among people with sleep apnea are so common that some sleep clinics give each sleep apnea patient a letter advising him not to drive until he has received treatment.

Accidents in the workplace can also be a major risk for people with sleep apnea and for their coworkers and clients. In the transportation industry, untreated sleep apnea is a public danger when it affects school bus drivers, truckers, airplane and ship pilots, railroad engineers, truck drivers, heavy equipment operators, and car pool drivers. People in these occupations who *ever* experience drowsiness on the job have an obligation either to identify and treat the cause of their drowsiness or to change occupations.

Once treatment for sleep apnea has begun, it is important for both health and safety to make sure that the treatment is actually having an effect. Feeling cured is not the same as being cured, as the following case illustrates.

Case Study. *Mr. Rodgers was diagnosed with moderately severe obstructive sleep apnea and underwent UPPP surgery. His snoring disappeared and he felt improved and no longer fell asleep at the wrong times. The surgeon recommended that he return to the sleep center for a retest, to* *see how much improvement had actually been achieved by the surgery. Mr. Rodgers refused to be retested because he was "absolutely sure" he was cured.*

Six months later Mr. Rodgers fell asleep while driving and wrecked his car. In retrospect he could recall occasionally feeling drowsy, even though he had improved significantly after surgery. A follow-up sleep study showed that he still had 50% of his sleep apnea. Further treatment resulted in full control of his symptoms.

If you suffer from excessive drowsiness, you owe it to yourself, your family, and others on the highway to refrain from driving until you have been tested to determine the cause of your problem and have begun effective treatment.

Breathing, Circulation, and Heart Problems

The cardiovascular (heart and circulatory system) and pulmonary (lung) effects of sleep apnea are very serious; over a period of years these effects become life-threatening. The cardiovascular effects of sleep apnea result in the nocturnal sudden death of approximately 2,000 to 3,000 people per year in the United States.[3] Let's look at some of the ways in which sleep apnea can damage people's health.

Low blood oxygen concentration during the night is typical in a person with sleep apnea. This is responsible for much of the long-term harm resulting from sleep apnea. With each apnea event the blood oxygen drops to an abnormally low level, depriving the body's cells of oxygen. The brain is particularly susceptible to low oxygen. If the low blood oxygen is severe and continued over a long period of time, it can unfavorably affect the brain. This may explain the changes in personality, memory, alertness, and coordination seen in people with sleep apnea.[4]

High blood pressure is one important cardiovascular effect of low blood oxygen. High blood pressure is seen in 35% to 50% of sleep apnea patients. Chronic high blood pressure results in enlargement of the heart, which is a risk factor for stroke and heart failure.[5]

The relationship between high blood pressure and sleep apnea is complicated and not well understood. Some people have significant improvement in their blood pressure once their sleep apnea is treated. Other people show little change because their high blood pressure has other causes.

Blood pressure may be indirectly improved when the treatment of sleep apnea allows the patient to lose weight and to enjoy regular exercise. Excess weight contributes to high blood pressure, and regular exercise can help to lower blood pressure.

Patients on high doses of blood pressure medications should make sure their doctors follow them carefully, after their sleep apnea is treated, to see if they need less medication. Otherwise, they may develop symptoms of *low* blood pressure, because their body no longer needs so much medication. Careful adjustments of medications are needed.

Sleep apnea contributes notably to a particular type of high blood pressure: unusually high pressure in the artery that carries blood from the right side of the heart to the lungs. This occurs mainly in people who have other health problems and already have low blood oxygen when they are awake. In time this condition can lead to enlargement of the right side of the heart and to fluid congestion in the lungs.[5–8]

Arrhythmia (abnormal heart rhythm) is seen in more than 90% of sleep apnea patients.[5] Abnormal slowing down of the heart, long pauses (more than two seconds), extra beats, and several other types of arrhythmias are associated with sleep apnea. People with sleep apnea are thought to run a higher than normal risk of sudden death from heart failure during the night, probably because of a fatal arrhythmia.[9]

The *operation of the lungs* is affected by changes in blood pressure, described earlier, that result from low blood oxygen. In addition, the low oxygen and high carbon dioxide concentrations in the blood result in abnormal blood chemistry. These changes in blood chemistry also disturb the functioning of the lungs.[10]

The combined damage from cardiopulmonary disturbances— abnormal blood pressure relationships in the heart and lungs, abnormal blood chemistry from too much carbon dioxide and too little oxygen, arrhythmias—is thought by most sleep specialists to be the greatest long-term danger to health from sleep apnea.[11]

SOCIAL AND PSYCHOLOGICAL EFFECTS

The fatigue, sleepiness, and medical complications that result from sleep apnea can virtually destroy a person's life.

Work performance is often profoundly undermined. People with sleep apnea may miss work frequently, arrive at work late, become drowsy or fall asleep at work, and have poor concentration and poor job performance. Their bosses and colleagues seldom understand their problems and often assume that the unusual behavior is due to drugs, alcohol, or serious personality problems. Promotions are missed, jobs are lost, promising careers are sidetracked.

Home life and social life also suffer. Studies have shown that married people with sleep apnea tend to become socially isolated and alienated from their partners and children. The fatigue and sleepiness of the sleep apnea sufferer lead him to participate less and less in family activities and relationships and to spend more and more time withdrawn or sleeping. Family life often begins to feel more like a burden than a source of support.[12]

His family may become critical of his inactivity, decreased work around the house, or negative and crabby attitude. The result is a puzzled, resentful, increasingly uncommunicative family. These problems may contribute to marital conflicts, child-raising difficulties, and divorce.

Psychological and memory problems are frequent results of sleep apnea. *Irritability* is common in people with moderate to severe sleep apnea, as are other personality changes, such as *depression*, and, less commonly, *memory impairment, confusion, anger,* and even *physical abuse. Loss of alertness and concentration* are not unusual. Patients with sleep apnea score lower than normal on tests for attention and concentration and on other tests of brain activity.[4]

The loss of mental acuity is usually so gradual that the person may not realize it is happening. First, he may find that reading is a chore, so he will read less. Then he may have trouble concentrating on other tasks or remembering words. It may not be until after his sleep apnea is under treatment and his mental facility begins to return that he realizes how much he had lost.

These neurologic changes are due both to poor sleep and to the abnormally low oxygen levels in the blood during sleep (discussed earlier).

To summarize, then, driving accidents may be the most immediate threat of death from sleep apnea. In the longer term, sleep apnea leads to life-threatening medical complications and psychological and social difficulties. Most of these consequences can be lessened or eliminated with treatment of the apnea. Treatment is discussed in Chapter 7.

DIAGNOSING AND TREATING SLEEP APNEA

Who Suffers from Sleep Apnea?

When does a person's tendency toward sleep apnea first arise? This is difficult to pinpoint, because sleep apnea results from the combination of several risk factors.

Sleep apnea can be found at all ages. In some people the tendency may be present at birth. Sleep apnea may be the later stage of a breathing disorder that begins early in life as a slight breathing instability—some part of the automatic breathing reflex that is slightly irregular.

A breathing instability is more likely to develop into sleep apnea when other important risk factors are present: obesity; an insensitive breathing reflex (see Chap. 3); a slight failure in coordination between the breathing muscles; an upper airway that is narrowed or obstructed by blockages in the nasal passages, large tonsils or adenoids, a large tongue, or a short lower jaw; and so on. Any of these factors may combine so that a slight breathing instability in a young person gradually evolves into a permanent abnormality in sleep breathing in an adult.[13]

The tendency to develop sleep apnea is probably inherited in some people. For example, a person may inherit an airway whose shape is easily obstructed. Or he may inherit a weak breathing response to carbon dioxide. Either one or a combination of several inherited factors may set the stage for a person to develop sleep apnea.[14]

Sex is a factor in the development of sleep apnea. Men are about three times more likely to have sleep apnea than women.[15] The reasons for this difference are unclear, but they may have to do with sexual differences in the structure of the airway or in muscle tone. The effects of sex hormones may also be a factor (e.g., progesterone in women versus testosterone in men).

Body weight is another factor. Obese people suffer a much higher incidence of sleep apnea than people of ideal weight. (See Chap. 8.)

In terms of age, sleep apnea is primarily a condition of middle age or older. This is true for several reasons. First, with age there is a loss of muscle tone in the throat during sleep. Second, when people do have untreated sleep apnea, the condition becomes worse as they grow older. Third, body weight tends to increase with age, beginning often after age 40. By the time the symptoms of sleep apnea are serious enough to attract medical attention, the person may be in his 40s or 50s and may be suffering from obesity, pulmonary complications, arrhythmia, even congestive heart failure. The average age of patients in one sleep clinic was reported to be 52.[16]

However, sleep apnea can occur at any age. Children can develop sleep apnea. In fact, now that tonsillectomies are less common than they used to be, sleep apnea is probably more prevalent in children than it was a generation ago. Children who have enlarged tonsils or adenoids or who are obese are the most likely to develop sleep apnea. (See Chap. 9 for information about apnea in infants and about SIDS and Chap. 10 for more about sleep apnea in older children.)

A number of drugs aggravate sleep apnea. These include alcohol, sedatives, hypnotic drugs ("sleeping pills"), and some heart medications (short-acting beta blockers, such as Inderal). (See the Appendix.)

Why Haven't You Heard of Sleep Apnea Before?

It has been estimated that 20 million Americans may have sleep apnea.[17] Among 30- to 60-year-olds, one of every four men and one of every ten women show some signs of sleep apnea. In a study of industrial workers in Israel, one out of every five was classified as having some degree of sleep apnea.[18] These are surprisingly large numbers of people, considering that a few years ago hardly anybody had ever heard of sleep apnea.

So if sleep apnea is this common, why haven't you heard about it before?

The answer is that sleep apnea has always been around, but it was not recognized by the medical community until recently.

One of the earliest descriptions of sleep apnea was published in 1877 by an observant medical man named W. H. Broadbent. He did not call the condition sleep apnea, but he described the two major types of apnea that today are called *obstructive* and *central* apnea.

During the late 1800s several additional reports were published about patients who suffered from abnormal daytime sleepiness and had difficulty breathing while asleep. In 1890 an early American neurologist and toxicologist named Silas Weir Mitchell wrote the first detailed accounts of a breathing disorder that occurred during sleep and began to unravel the mystery of what causes sleep apnea.

Unfortunately for those suffering from sleep apnea, bacteria came into vogue soon after that. Medical attention focused upon sleep diseases that were caused by microbes, such as sleeping sickness, and little interest or credence was given to other kinds of sleep disorders or their causes. As a result, much of what had been learned or suggested about sleep disorders lapsed into neglect.

It was not until the 1950s that several groups of scientists began to make careful observations of actual sleeping people. They developed an electronic technique for measuring and studying sleep, called *polysomnography*. (See Chap. 6.) Using this technique, they began to discover interesting things about what goes on during sleep. They learned, for example, that sleep is not at all a time of peaceful inactivity. This unexpected discovery stimulated an explosion of interest in sleep research and intensified the quest for a better understanding of sleep, both normal and abnormal.

It soon became apparent that events during sleep can profoundly affect a person's health. As explained by William Dement, one of the leaders in this field: "It is possible for individuals to be entirely normal awake and deathly ill asleep."[19] Thus a new field of medicine, *sleep disorders medicine*, began to take shape.

In the past 15 years sleep researchers have learned how to recognize the signs of various abnormal sleep conditions—sleep apnea, narcolepsy, nocturnal myoclonus, idiopathic CNS hypersomnolence, and others—that previously had been difficult or impossible to diagnose. Physicians are becoming better informed and are beginning to diagnose sleep apnea in patients who previously might simply have been treated for "insomnia," heart problems, or some other symptom.

Confirming the Diagnosis and Treating Sleep Apnea

Once you have been given a tentative diagnosis of sleep apnea, an all-night sleep test should be arranged. Proper testing for sleep disorders is important. Several different sleep disorders have superficial similarities to sleep apnea and might be confused with sleep apnea if testing were not done properly. An incorrect diagnosis, leading to incorrect treatment, can be a serious error. For example, medications that are often prescribed for narcolepsy or insomnia can actually worsen sleep apnea, so a correct diagnosis is very important.

Narcolepsy is a sleep disorder in which people have irresistible "sleep attacks" at inappropriate times, somewhat as in sleep apnea. However, narcolepsy is a distinct neurologic disorder with other characteristic symptoms (cataplexy, sleep paralysis, and hypnagogic hallucinations) not found in sleep apnea.

Insomnia is sometimes confused with sleep apnea. Insomnia has numerous causes, and only a few people who have insomnia also have sleep apnea.

Two other sleep disorders sometimes occur alone or along with sleep apnea. These are *periodic leg movement* (PLM, or nocturnal myoclonus) and *restless leg syndrome*. Again, appropriate testing by an experienced sleep disorders specialist will avoid confusing one sleep disorder with another.

An overnight sleep test will:

✦ Confirm whether you actually have sleep apnea.

✦ Determine the type of sleep apnea, which must be known in order to select the appropriate treatment; and

✦ Rule out other sleep disorders.

Chapters 4 through 7 of this book will take you through the processes of diagnosis and treatment of sleep apnea. Chapter 4 describes the three types of sleep apnea. Chapter 5 discusses some of the difficulties in diagnosing sleep apnea. Testing for sleep apnea is described in Chapter 6. Treatment methods are discussed in Chapter 7.

Chapter 3 is included for those readers who would like a better understanding of sleep and the causes of sleep apnea.

Summary

❖ *Sleep apnea is not yet widely recognized by family doctors.*

❖ *Sleep apnea can occur at any age but is most common in middle age, particularly among men and people who are obese.*

❖ *Sleep apnea is treatable.*

❖ *Sleep apnea can devastate a person's career, wreak havoc on family and social life, and cause psychological and memory problems.*

❖ *Sleep apnea can be life-threatening if not treated. It results in:*

Auto accidents.

Workplace accidents.

Abnormal blood chemistry.

High blood pressure.

Arrhythmia (irregular heartbeat).

Other heart complications.

Lung complications.

Loss of alertness, memory, concentration.

Death.

➤ ➤ ➤ ➤ ➤ 3 ➤ ➤ ➤ ➤ ➤

Normal Sleep, Snoring, and the Development of Sleep Apnea

This chapter is for the reader who likes to understand how things work. Not everyone will be interested in finding out what happens inside his or her body to cause sleep apnea. But anyone can understand the causes of sleep apnea, and that understanding will help make it seem less frightening or mysterious.

Understanding the cause of sleep apnea will also give you a better grasp of the kinds of treatment that are used and of the importance of carrying through with long-term treatment. You will be better equipped to discuss treatment options with your doctor and to play an active role in choosing the most appropriate treatment.

SLEEP, NORMAL AND ABNORMAL

To understand the causes and results of sleep apnea, it helps to know a little about what happens during a normal night's sleep.

Why Do We Sleep?

Nobody knows exactly why we sleep. At one time people thought that sleep was just a rest period for our brains. Then

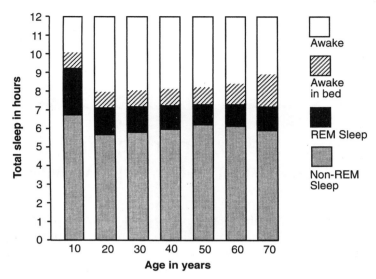

FIG. 3.1. Changes in sleep over a lifetime.

polysomnography was developed. This technology allows scientists to make electrical recordings of brain activities during sleep. Scientists were surprised to discover that brains are anything but idle during the night.

Some theories suggest that we sleep to overcome body fatigue. Our bodies do seem to overcome fatigue during sleep, but studies have shown that it is our brain, not our muscles, that requires sleep in order to feel rested and function normally.

How much sleep do we need? Actually, there is no "normal" amount of sleep that is right for everybody. The amount of sleep a person needs is a very individual matter and also varies according to age and circumstances (see Fig. 3.1).

It used to be said, for example, that babies needed 21 hours of sleep per day, but now it is known that the amount of sleep they need varies a great deal from infant to infant. Sixteen-year-olds seem to need around ten or 11 hours, and this decreases to about eight hours for an average adult. But there are cases of healthy, alert adults who do fine on four hours of sleep. The record for habitually short sleep seems to be about three hours per night.[1] No one has ever been documented to need *no* sleep.

What happens if people are experimentally deprived of sleep for several days? They have periodic bouts of drowsiness, when their built-in biological clock tries to get them to go to sleep. They suffer a gradual, increasing loss of concentration and mental sharpness. They may become irritable and disoriented and may have dreamlike hallucinations. Reactions become slow and erratic. Beyond that the effects of sleep deprivation seem generally to depend upon an individual's personality. For example, the person who is prone to mental breakdown may show signs of disturbed behavior if he is deprived of sleep for several days. Another person may behave in a relatively normal manner.

Clearly, sleep deprivation is not fatal. In fact, it is prescribed as a treatment for certain types of depression. However, long-term lack of sufficient sleep does interfere with normal behavior and performance.

To be at our best, each of us needs a certain *quantity* of sleep every night. If we do not get enough sleep, we tend to build up a sleep "debt." This leads to a tendency to feel drowsy during the day and to fall asleep more readily.

But the quantity of sleep we get is not the whole story. Equally important is the *quality* of our sleep. Does it come in large, continuous blocks, or is it fragmented into short naps? Do we get enough "deep" sleep?

The quality of our sleep is related to a series of sleep stages that the brain passes through during the night. These are described in the next section.

In people with sleep apnea, sleep is broken up by numerous awakenings during the night, reducing the quantity of sleep they obtain. In addition, the numerous awakenings break up the structure, or continuity, of their sleep. They miss out on some of the normal stages of sleep. This lowers the quality of their sleep. Thus sleep apnea affects both the quantity and the quality of sleep.

Let's look a little more closely at what goes on in your brain while you are sleeping.

The Stages of Normal Sleep

After you go to sleep, the activities of your brain and body settle into fairly predictable patterns. Sleep researchers have discovered that there are two kinds of sleep: REM sleep and non-REM (or NREM) sleep. REM stands for *Rapid Eye Movement*, and in a moment you will see why. REM and NREM sleep alternate with each other during the night.

NREM sleep is "quiet" sleep. Your breathing and brain activity are slow and regular, and your body is quiet and relaxed. You may dream, but the dreams will be more thoughtlike than emotional.

REM sleep, in contrast, is "active" sleep. There are active changes in your physiology during REM sleep. For example, your breathing becomes irregular, alternating between slow and fast. You may stop breathing every now and then for several seconds. Your body temperature rises, and the blood circulation in your brain increases. The large muscles of your body—your leg and arm muscles—actually become paralyzed: you *cannot* move them, except for little twitches of your face and fingertips. But your eye muscles become very active and move your eyes back and forth as if they were watching a ping-pong match. This, of course, is the rapid eye movement that led to the term *REM sleep*. Much, but not all, of your dreaming occurs during REM sleep. The most vivid, intense, emotional dreams almost always occur during REM sleep.

A typical night's sleep begins with "quiet" NREM sleep. There are four stages of NREM sleep, which progress from light to heavy sleep. Then, rather abruptly, about 70 to 90 minutes from the beginning of sleep, your sleep lightens from its deepest level to reach the first "active" REM period. That first REM sleep period usually lasts about ten minutes. It ends when sleep shifts back into lighter Stage 2 NREM sleep. Then sleep begins to deepen and the cycle starts all over again.

This cycle takes about 90 minutes and repeats itself throughout the night. Early in the night the REM periods in the cycle are shorter. During the second half of the night, REM periods

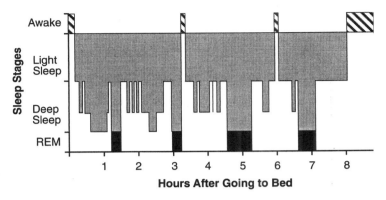

FIG 3.2. A typical night's sleep of a normal young adult. Notice how the sleep pattern shifts from stage to stage during the night.

become longer, sometimes as long as 60 minutes, separated only by short periods of Stage 2 NREM sleep (see Fig. 3.2).

The total amount of REM sleep during the night varies with age. Newborn babies spend about half of their sleeping time in REM sleep. By adulthood, REM sleep has decreased to about a quarter of our total sleep time.

We all seem to need REM sleep, although nobody knows exactly why. The need may be related to REM dreaming, during which we seem to "process" the emotion-laden experiences of waking life.

In any case, our bodies appear to have an automatic mechanism that "tries" to obtain the normal amount of REM sleep for us. When people are deprived of REM sleep and then allowed to sleep normally, they usually experience several nights of what is called *REM rebound.* In REM rebound, people spend an especially long time in REM sleep. They often remember dreaming more and having more vivid and often scarier dreams than normal. It is as if their bodies sense that they have been deprived of REM sleep and are catching up on what was missed.

As you will see later in this chapter, people with sleep apnea are often deprived of the normal amount of REM sleep.

Normal Breathing During Sleep

Breathing Centers and Reflexes

Your breathing movements during sleep are controlled by automatic reflexes. These reflexes are driven by nerve sensors, which constantly monitor the chemistry of your blood and send signals to the breathing centers of your brain. These centers, in turn, send signals to your breathing muscles to regulate how fast and how powerfully you need to breathe at any particular time (see Fig. 3.3). This regulatory activity of the brain's breathing centers is one of the factors in the development of sleep apnea.

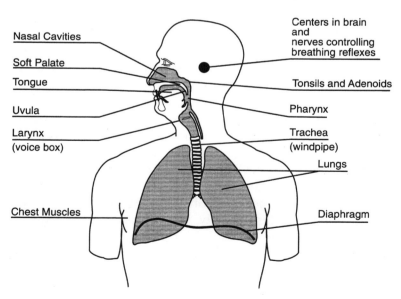

FIG. 3.3. The parts of the body that are involved in the breathing reflex.

Sensors and "Set Points"

One group of nerve sensors for monitoring your blood chemistry is in your *carotid bodies*. The carotid bodies, located in the carotid arteries in your neck, sense the amount of oxygen in the blood that is on its way to your brain. The carotid bodies respond to low levels of oxygen in your blood. But even though oxygen is essential for life, particularly for your brain cells, these sensors are not the most important ones for your breathing reflex.

A more powerful set of sensors is in a deep and primitive part of your brain called the *medulla*. These sensors detect increases in the carbon dioxide in your cerebrospinal fluid (the fluid that bathes your brain and spinal cord). Carbon dioxide, your body's waste gas, is produced as the oxygen in your body is used up. A high concentration of carbon dioxide in your cerebrospinal fluid signals that your body needs to breathe. When you breathe, you exhale carbon dioxide and immediately inhale fresh oxygen.

The particular concentration of carbon dioxide that triggers these sensors can be called the *set point*. Whenever the carbon dioxide concentration rises high enough to reach the set point, the breathing reflex is activated. The oxygen sensors probably work in a similar way, but their set points are not nearly as sensitive during sleep.

The set points that trigger your breathing reflexes can move up and down, depending on a number of factors, including whether you are awake or asleep. During sleep the set points do not have to be as sensitive to low oxygen and high carbon dioxide as they do when you are awake, because your sleeping body needs less oxygen, your breathing is more shallow, and the air in your lungs is exchanged less vigorously. So as you pass from waking to sleeping to waking, the set points cycle up and down.[2]

Even during sleep the set points seem to change. For example, during REM sleep the breathing responses become less sensitive. More carbon dioxide is tolerated and the oxygen concentration can sometimes drop extremely low during REM sleep before the breathing reflexes finally are triggered.[2]

The sensitivity of the set points is another factor in the development of sleep apnea.

Breathing Muscles

The movements of breathing require the use of muscle groups in a number of places: the diaphragm, the rib cage (the intercostal and other muscles that attach to the ribs), the soft palate, the tongue, the upper and lower pharynx (the throat area behind the mouth), and the larynx (voice box). When breathing is normal, the actions of these assorted muscles are carefully coordinated. For example, when you inhale, your rib muscles contract, your tongue muscles automatically stabilize the position of your tongue, and your soft palate muscles become taut to hold your airway open.

The coordination among these various muscle groups during breathing is another factor in the development of sleep apnea (see Fig. 3.4).

Snoring

Snoring occurs when your soft palate (the back part of the roof of your mouth) vibrates. A number of factors cause this. During sleep the muscle tone in your tongue and soft palate tends to decrease. They become more relaxed and can collapse together. This contributes to snoring.

Other soft tissues, such as tonsils and tongue, can produce sounds that add to or change the quality of the snoring.

The position of the sleeper affects the amount of snoring. Lying on your back allows your tongue to fall back toward your throat and block your airway; so you are more likely to snore when you are lying on your back.

Anything that obstructs your airway will also contribute to snoring. For example, you are more likely to snore if you have large adenoids or a large tongue or if your nasal passages are swollen from a cold or allergies.

Age is also a factor. Older people tend to snore more because muscle tone tends to decrease with age.

Other factors also aggravate snoring; alcoholic beverages, certain medications, and sheer physical exhaustion may be associated with heavy snoring.

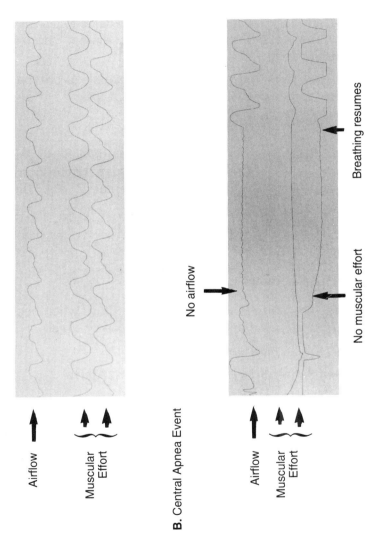

A. Normal Sleep

Airflow

Muscular
Effort

B. Central Apnea Event

No airflow

No muscular effort

Breathing resumes

Airflow

Muscular
Effort

FIG. 3.4. Typical patterns of breathing, showing airflow and movement of breathing muscles, **(A)** during normal sleep and **(B)** in a central apnea event, in which the breathing reflexes do not operate normally.

Mere snoring, by itself, is not the same as sleep apnea. Many people snore without having the complete interruptions of breathing and sleep that are the signs of sleep apnea. Light or occasional snoring that does not interrupt breathing is not a health threat, although it can be a terrific annoyance to a sleeping partner. The solutions to harmless occasional snoring include the following:

✤ Sleep on your side. You can train yourself to sleep on your side using a sleep position monitor. (See Chapter 7.)

✤ Avoid alcohol before going to bed.

✤ Check with your doctor to see whether any medication you are taking (either by prescription or over the counter) may be aggravating the snoring. (See Chapter 7 and the Appendix.)

✤ If nasal congestion is a problem for you, ask your doctor about an antihistamine to reduce swelling.

✤ Decrease your body weight.

✤ For the sleeping partner, wear soft foam earplugs when necessary. They are available from industrial safety stores.

When Simple Snoring Turns into Sleep Apnea

In some people the loss of muscle tone in the tongue and throat is accompanied by a number of other factors, discussed earlier in this chapter: an instability in the breathing reflexes, a structural narrowing of the airway, or a lack of coordination among the breathing muscles.

In these people slight or occasional snoring may gradually develop into the heavy, more violent snoring that indicates sleep apnea. This process often begins in adolescence with heavy snoring and occasional, short clusters of apnea events. Gradually, the picture may change to heavier snoring with longer sequences of nonbreathing. Later in adulthood the pattern may evolve into obstructive apnea events that occur throughout nearly the whole night, with great disturbances in the structure of sleep, fluctuations in oxygen content of the blood, and day-time drowsiness.[3]

In some older people who have never had trouble with sleep apnea the loss of muscle tone that occurs with age is enough to trigger the development of sleep apnea.

The reason why snoring may progress to sleep apnea in some people and not in others depends on the sum of all the factors we have described here: breathing reflexes, structure of the airway, muscle coordination, and inherited tendencies.

Summary

❖ *The most important aspects of sleep are the following:*

  The quantity of sleep.

  The quality of sleep.

  The amount of REM (rapid eye movement) sleep.

❖ *Sleep apnea interferes with all three of these.*

❖ *An abnormality in the breathing reflex during sleep can contribute to the development of sleep apnea.*

❖ *Snoring is caused by loss of muscle tone in the tongue and throat.*

❖ *Most of the sounds of typical snoring are caused by the vibration of the soft palate.*

❖ *Snoring in which breathing does not stop is probably harmless. You may be able to decrease or eliminate this type of snoring by following suggestions in this chapter.*

❖ *Snoring in which breathing stops is a symptom of sleep apnea.*

➤ ➤ ➤ ➤ ➤ 4 ➤ ➤ ➤ ➤ ➤

What Causes Sleep Apnea?

A TYPICAL MIXED APNEA EVENT

*M*r. *Kennedy crawls into bed and turns out the light. He immediately falls asleep and begins to snore softly. His wife stuffs earplugs into her ears and wills herself to fall asleep quickly, before her husband really starts to snore. She reaches over and shakes his elbow.*

"Roll over," she reminds him.

He complies, turns onto his side, and resumes his snoring.

Over the next few minutes the sound of each snore becomes louder, more prolonged, more emphatic. Then all at once the room is silent. The snoring has stopped.

Mr. Kennedy is lying very still. In fact, he is not breathing.

What has happened? The breathing center in Mr. Kennedy's brain has stopped working. As a result, the breathing muscles in his diaphragm and chest receive no signals. They stop moving. (This is a sign of *central apnea*.)

When breathing movements stop, oxygen cannot get into the lungs, nor can carbon dioxide get out. Consequently, the oxygen concentration in Mr. Kennedy's blood begins to drop and the concentration of carbon dioxide increases.

Mr. Kennedy is slowly suffocating.

Eventually, extreme concentrations of oxygen and carbon dioxide stimulate his nerve sensors. (The further their set point is from "normal," the longer it will take for this to happen. See Chap. 3.) When Mr. Kennedy's sensors finally respond, they tell his brain's breathing center to start working again. His breathing center again sends signals to the breathing muscles, and once again he begins to make breathing movements.

However, Mr. Kennedy's problems are not over; even though the chest muscles have begun to work, no air is going in or out of his lungs. This is because the airway in his throat collapsed shut when he first stopped breathing. His chest heaves in and out now, even shaking the mattress with the force of the muscle contractions; but his throat is closed, so there still is no actual movement of air in and out. (This is a sign of *obstructive apnea*.)

Mr. Kennedy may struggle for a breath of air for as long as a minute, or even longer. Meanwhile, the oxygen supply in his body is running out and the carbon dioxide is accumulating.

Fortunately for Mr. Kennedy and the rest of our species, we all have a primitive, fail-safe, emergency arousal response. It awakens us at just such times as this and keeps us from suffocating during sleep. When Mr. Kennedy's arousal response finally is triggered, he wakes up. His body jerks and he gasps for air with a series of loud, snorting breaths, sucking oxygen into his lungs like a diver returning from the depths. This is the explosive snoring that is typical of sleep apnea.

In just a few seconds fresh air pours into his lungs and the oxygen concentration in his blood reaches nearly normal, the carbon dioxide is expelled, and he returns to sleep. The arousal has been so brief that Mr. Kennedy is not aware of being awakened. But the normal pattern of his sleep has been broken. People with severe apnea may never reach deep sleep; they have very fragmented REM sleep because of the constant arousals. Thus throughout the night it is the deepest sleep that is most disturbed.

A short while after Mr. Kennedy returns to sleep—perhaps two minutes, perhaps five—the whole process will repeat itself.

Mr. Kennedy is an example of a person who has mixed apnea, a combination of central sleep apnea and obstructive sleep apnea.

THE THREE TYPES OF SLEEP APNEA

There are three kinds of sleep apnea, classified according to their causes: central sleep apnea, obstructive sleep apnea, and mixed apnea. Some sleep researchers believe that the distinctions, at least between central and obstructive apnea, are very clear; other sleep experts feel that the differences are blurred.

The distinction between central, obstructive, and mixed apnea is important because of their respective causes. The cause of the apnea determines treatment. Let's look at the cause of each type of sleep apnea.

Central Apnea

Pure central apnea is the least common of the three types of sleep apnea. In *central apnea* the cause of the breathing problem is in the brain, or central nervous system; thus the term "central apnea." In a person with central apnea the respiratory center in the brain that controls breathing (described in Chap. 3) may simply stop working during sleep. It fails to signal the chest muscles to make breathing movements. Sleep researchers believe this may happen for a number of reasons, all related to some disorder in the breathing reflex. The disorder may be an inherited neurologic problem or a neuromuscular disorder that arises later in life, such as polio or ALS (amyotrophic lateral sclerosis, or Lou Gehrig's disease).

A person with pure central apnea has great difficulty sleeping and breathing at the same time. As soon as he drops off to sleep, he stops breathing (Fig. 4.1). When his emergency arousal response takes over, he awakens with a start and a gasp. In severe central apnea the person may get very little sleep at all. This is an extremely distressing condition that can last for many years before it is correctly diagnosed.

Another form of central apnea is sometimes seen in people who have a psychological problem called *sleep onset anxiety.* People with sleep onset anxiety are panicky about falling asleep. This causes them to breathe quickly and heavily, resulting in a decrease in the carbon dioxide in their blood. When they do fall

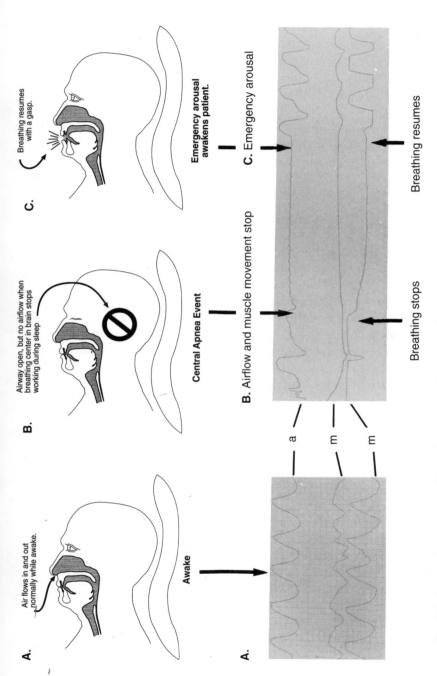

Fig. 4.1. A central apnea event. The polysomnograph tracings show the airflow in and out of the airway (a) and the movement of the breathing muscles (m). **A:** Normal breathing while awake. **B:** During sleep, breathing movements and airflow stop. **C:** Emergency arousal awakens the person and he resumes breathing with a gasp.

asleep, the low carbon dioxide fails to trigger their breathing reflex for a long time. Consequently, they end up having a central apnea event and awakening to breathe.

Typically, the main complaint of a person with central apnea is that he doesn't get enough sleep. He may describe his problem as "insomnia." The reason for his complaint, of course, is his frequent awakenings during the night. However, not all people with insomnia have sleep apnea. In fact, only about 5% of insomniacs show even slight signs of sleep apnea.

In a person with pure central apnea, obstruction of the airway is not usually a problem. However, research suggests that sometimes obstructive apnea can trigger central apnea.[1] In these cases if the airway obstruction is treated, the central apnea may disappear.

The long-term effects of central apnea are similar to the effects of obstructive apnea: enlargement of the heart, lung complications, and heart failure.

Drug therapy is a promising method of treating central apnea. Other treatments might involve surgery, if there are airway obstructions, and possibly the use of a nighttime ventilating device. Pacemakers for the diaphragm have also been developed and may eventually be an acceptable treatment for central apnea. (See Chap. 7 for more on treatment of sleep apnea.)

Obstructive Sleep Apnea

In obstructive sleep apnea the upper airway is blocked during sleep by the tissue of the soft palate, throat, and tongue. In Chapter 3 we explained that this blockage can result from a combination of anatomic factors and irregularities in the breathing reflex.

Unlike the patient with central apnea, who simply stops breathing, the person with obstructive sleep apnea struggles to breathe against the obstructed airway (Fig. 4.2). His chest moves in and out, but because of the blockage, the air cannot flow into or out of his lungs. Finally, his oxygen concentration drops, as Mr. Kennedy's did, to the point where his arousal reflex causes him to breathe. He awakens with a loud, gasping, snorting sound.

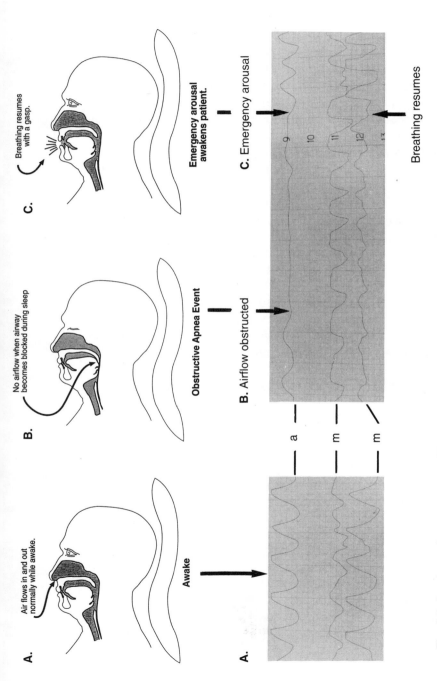

Fig. 4.2. An obstructive apnea event. The polysomnograph recording shows airflow in and out of the airway (a) and the movements of the breathing muscles (m). **A:** Normal breathing while awake. **B:** During sleep the airway collapses and becomes obstructed. The breathing muscles continue to move, but no air can flow into the airway. **C:** Emergency arousal awakens the person, and he resumes breathing with a gasp.

People with obstructive apnea may have one or more anatomic abnormalities associated with their upper airway: the passages in their nose and pharynx (throat) (Fig. 4.3). Such abnormalities can be seen in head x-ray images of many people with obstructive sleep apnea.[2]

In the nose the abnormal structure may be a deviated nasal septum or chronic swelling of the nasal passages as a result of allergies.

In the upper pharynx, obstructions may include enlarged tonsils or adenoids, an extra-long or fleshy soft palate, or a large uvula (the fleshy tab that dangles in the back of your throat.) In the lower pharynx the problem might be a large tongue, a tongue that is located unusually far back or far down, an unusually small airway opening, a short lower jaw, or a short neck.[2]

Any one of these structural features, or a combination of them, can help cause obstructive sleep apnea (Fig. 4.3).

Body weight is often a factor in the development of obstructive apnea. One-half to three-fourths of patients with obstructive sleep apnea are more than 15% over their ideal weight.[3]

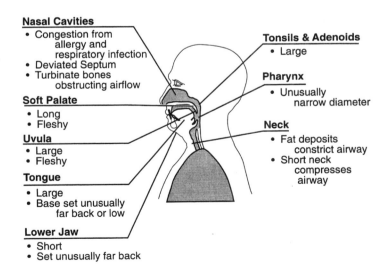

Nasal Cavities
- Congestion from allergy and respiratory infection
- Deviated Septum
- Turbinate bones obstructing airflow

Soft Palate
- Long
- Fleshy

Uvula
- Large
- Fleshy

Tongue
- Large
- Base set unusually far back or low

Lower Jaw
- Short
- Set unusually far back

Tonsils & Adenoids
- Large

Pharynx
- Unusually narrow diameter

Neck
- Fat deposits constrict airway
- Short neck compresses airway

Fig. 4.3. Possible sources of airway obstructions in people with obstructive apnea.

Obstructive sleep apnea is common in overweight people for a couple of reasons. First of all, people who are carrying extra weight usually have fatty deposits within the throat tissue, which narrow the upper airway. Second, in some heavy people the extra weight on the abdomen changes the way their stomach and chest muscles work, alters the operation of their breathing reflexes, and contributes to the development of apnea. (See Chap. 8 for more on obesity and sleep apnea.)

Age is also a factor in obstructive sleep apnea, as already mentioned, because the shape and muscle tone of a person's upper airway tend to change with age. Many people have no sign of obstructive sleep apnea when they're younger but develop it in their 50s or 60s. (See Chap. 11 for more about age and sleep apnea.)

Sex is also a factor. Obstructive sleep apnea is about three times more prevalent among men.

Obstructive sleep apnea is treated by attempting to remove whatever is blocking the airway. This can be accomplished by means of a breathing device, through surgery, and sometimes by both. If obesity is a factor, weight loss usually helps, if it can be maintained. (See Chap. 7 for treatment of sleep apnea.)

When a physician is seeking the cause, it is extremely important to determine very carefully which of these many factors are contributing to the obstructive apnea, so that the most effective treatment can be chosen.

Mixed Apnea

Mixed apnea is a combination of central and obstructive apnea. Most people with sleep apnea probably have some form of mixed apnea. In fact, some sleep researchers believe that most, if not all, obstructive sleep apnea has a central apnea component and that some abnormality in the breathing reflex in the brain usually accompanies the development of obstructive apnea.

Others interpret the cause and effect that occur in mixed apnea a little differently. They point out that as a person gasps and recovers from an obstructive apnea event, he typically "overbreathes," and this results in an unusually low level of carbon dioxide in his blood. In turn, this lower carbon dioxide is enough to trigger a central apnea event, thereby producing mixed apnea. The more severe the obstructive apnea, the more severe the "overbreathing" is likely to be and the more obvious the central apnea component could be expected to be.

In any case, whatever the actual cause and effect in mixed apnea, the obstructive apnea is usually treated first. So you could say that, for treatment purposes, most mixed apnea is obstructive apnea. Once the breathing obstruction is treated, the central apnea will often disappear, or at least lessen to the point where it does not require treatment.

Summary

❖ *Snoring in which breathing stops is a symptom of sleep apnea.*

❖ *There are three kinds of sleep apnea:*

  Central apnea, the least common, originates in the brain.

  Obstructive sleep apnea is caused by a blockage in the airway.

  Mixed apnea, the most common, is a combination of central and obstructive apnea.

❖ *The choice of treatment depends on the kind of apnea.*

Problems and Pitfalls of Identifying Sleep Apnea

SEEKING THE CORRECT DIAGNOSIS

The first step in treating any medical problem is, of course, the correct diagnosis. To diagnose sleep apnea correctly, two important questions need to be answered:

1. Is this condition actually sleep apnea, or is it some other disorder?

2. Is sleep apnea the only disorder present, or are other conditions present that will complicate both the sleep apnea and the treatment?

Correct diagnosis of sleep apnea can be difficult for several reasons. Sleep apnea often is confused with a number of other sleep disorders, such as narcolepsy, insomnia, restless leg syndrome, or periodic leg movement. Or the opposite can occur: other disorders (heart conditions, breathing problems, seizure disorders) can be misdiagnosed as sleep apnea. Finally, sleep apnea can be both hidden and aggravated by other factors, such as certain medications (sedatives, hypnotics, and beta blockers), alcohol, heart disease, obesity. For these reasons it is important for someone with suspected sleep apnea to be thoroughly tested by a sleep specialist. Incorrect or mistaken treatment can be harmful.

Difficulties in Recognizing Sleep Apnea

Diagnosis is perhaps the most challenging aspect of sleep apnea. Unlike other diseases, sleep apnea does not allow the patient to be of much help to the diagnostician. The patient seldom recognizes the nature of the problem and cannot describe the most obvious symptoms because he is asleep when they occur.

Sleep specialists use *polysomnography* to confirm the diagnosis of sleep apnea and other sleep disorders. Polysomnography is the electronic measurement of sleep. It consists of hooking a patient up to electronic monitors, recording the patient's physiological signals on paper during a full night's sleep, and then analyzing the recording of the electronic signals. Until these tools were available, sleep apnea went unrecognized.

Appropriately used, polysomnographic testing can distinguish between sleep disorders and other conditions and can measure their severity. Polysomnography is described in detail in the next chapter.

Even with these modern tools, however, sleep apnea is occasionally misdiagnosed. Inappropriate sleep testing can lead to incorrect diagnosis and treatment. Tests must be done according to established standards; otherwise, the test results may be faulty. For example, testing for sleep apnea by means of daytime naps or a partial night's sleep may give a false picture: Daytime sleep is qualitatively different from nighttime sleep, and sleep apnea often is worse during the second half of the night, when most of REM sleep occurs.

Another reason why sleep apnea has been difficult to diagnose is that most medical people are not very familiar with the condition. Only in the 1980s has sleep apnea begun to be recognized as a specific sleep/breathing disorder with characteristic causes and symptoms. It is still best understood by sleep specialists. Even today the average medical student receives only about 24 minutes of instruction on sleep disorders during his/her entire medical education.[1]

Unless your doctor is a recent graduate of one of the few medical schools that teaches about sleep disorders, his only contact with the field may be the medical literature, which contains an occasional article about sleep disorders. And reading about sleep apnea is not the same as recognizing the symptoms in a patient. The diagnostic routines that most doctors learn in medical school *never* prompt them to look for the symptoms of sleep apnea.

So a typical sequence of treatment begins when a physician fails to recognize the sleep apnea and attempts to treat the symptoms. Complaints of snoring, excessive daytime sleepiness (EDS), unexplained fatigue, and/or "insomnia" should be clear signals of possible sleep apnea. Instead these symptoms often are treated with drugs, such as stimulants or sleeping medications, and the underlying sleep apnea is missed or even aggravated, sometimes for many years.

The condition may become severe enough that heart and lung complications appear, as in the case of Mr. Allen (mentioned in Chap. 1). Even then many physicians will continue to treat the symptoms, without suspecting an underlying sleep/breathing disorder as the cause.

The difficulties in diagnosing sleep apnea have led to an enormous amount of frustration. Sick people go from doctor to doctor, for years, tortured by sleep apnea, desperately seeking an answer. People have died, and many more have reached the brink of death, before a chance encounter (a spouse, a friend, a news article, a change of physicians) finally has brought them to a sleep center for proper testing and a clear diagnosis of sleep apnea.

Avoiding Misdiagnosis: Ten Rules

The following are ten rules for avoiding misdiagnosis:

> **1. Select an accredited sleep center and be evaluated by a physician who has specialized in sleep disorders.**

How can you know if the sleep center and the physician are accredited? Call the American Sleep Disorders Association (ASDA) in Rochester, Minnesota (507-287-6006), and ask them for the nearest accredited sleep specialist or sleep center. Or you can ask whether a particular sleep lab has been accredited by the ASDA or whether a particular physician is a specialist in sleep disorders. (See also Chap. 12.)

There are many good sleep labs that are not accredited. If you live in an area of the country that has no accredited sleep centers, you may have to choose one that is not. In that case, call your state medical society and ask if they can refer you to a pulmonologist (lung specialist) who is familiar with treating sleep apnea. Many nonaccredited sleep labs are operated by pulmonologists or other physicians who have had training in the treatment of sleep apnea.

However, accreditation is the consumer's best signpost for locating a competent sleep center. A physician earns accreditation in sleep disorders medicine by passing a rigorous two-day examination. To be sure you are being treated by someone who is a certified sleep expert, ask the following question: "Have you passed the examination for sleep specialists given by the American Board of Sleep Medicine?" If you are hesitant about asking your doctor this question directly, you can telephone his office and ask his receptionist the question. If she does not know the answer, ask her to find out and call you back.

Case Study. *Mr. Woods was seen at his neighborhood hospital and told that he needed a sleep study. He was assured that the hospital had a "sleep lab" and that a "sleep expert" would diagnose his problem. In the hospital he was told he had central sleep apnea and was discouraged to learn that not much could be done for him.*

Later Mr. Woods was studied in an accredited sleep center, where he was found to have idiopathic CNS hypersomnolence, not central apnea. He also had mild sleep apnea, but it was obstructive rather than central. With medications for his idiopathic CNS hypersomnolence, he was able to return to work, and with weight loss the obstructive apnea disappeared.

> ## 2. Be sure that your sleep study is performed at night, or during your usual sleep hours.

If you are told to "stay awake all night and then come into the laboratory in the morning to have your sleep test," find another sleep center.

If you are a shift worker and are accustomed to sleeping during the day, either have your study during the day or switch back to sleeping at night for at least three nights prior to going into the lab for a sleep study at night.

Case Study. Mr. Daly was told to stay up all night and then come into the sleep lab to have a sleep study. He slept poorly in the lab, and after three hours had to end the study because he couldn't sleep any longer. He was diagnosed as having some sleep apnea and told to lose weight.

Later he was restudied properly in a nighttime sleep test at an accredited sleep center. He was found to have severe sleep apnea, particularly during the last four hours of the night, which the earlier sleep study had missed because it did not examine Mr. Daly during his usual sleep hours.

Appropriate treatment included not only weight loss but UPPP surgery and the use of CPAP. (See Chap. 7.) With treatment Mr. Daly improved remarkably and eventually was even able to discontinue CPAP.

> ## 3. If you are sleepy while driving and working, be sure that, on the day following your nighttime sleep study, a Multiple Sleep Latency Test (MSLT) is performed.

An MSLT will establish the severity of your daytime sleepiness. It will also help rule out other causes of sleepiness (for example, other sleep disorders) and provide a baseline to refer to if fatigue and sleepiness continue after the apnea has been treated.

Case Study. Ms. Jones snored badly and had been tired for years. She was sleepy driving and couldn't stay awake during her favorite operas. She went to a "sleep lab" and was told she needed UPPP surgery.

After surgery she was pleased that she no longer snored, felt better, and was not sleepy while driving. However, she still felt tired. She was told that her trouble was due to stress and boredom.

She was restudied at an accredited sleep center and her Multiple Sleep Latency Test showed that despite the surgery, she still had most of her sleep apnea. It also uncovered a second major sleep disorder that previously had been missed: narcolepsy.

> **4. Be sure that you have had a recent thorough physical examination and laboratory studies, preferably with your own physician, who knows your past health problems and has all your records available.**

This will avoid duplication of tests.

Case Study. *Mr. Roberts was told that sleep apnea was the cause of his snoring and progressive fatigue. He had gained weight, so he was put on a weight loss program and referred to a surgeon for UPPP surgery.*

He obtained a second opinion at an accredited sleep center, and a physical exam found that he had low thyroid activity. Treatment eliminated his fatigue. He quickly lost the extra weight, which had also been caused by his thyroid disorder, and his apnea then disappeared.

> **5. Be sure you have a thorough examination of your throat, preferably by an ear, nose, and throat specialist (also known as an ENT specialist or otolaryngologist) who is experienced with sleep apnea.**

Case Study. *Mr. Wilson had been told by his doctor that he probably had sleep apnea, but the doctor wouldn't refer him to a sleep center unless he lost weight. Six months later Mr. Wilson felt worse and obtained a referral from another physician.*

He was found to have mild apnea, and an ENT physician examined his throat and found a cancer narrowing his lower throat area. Mr. Wilson then realized he had been having a little trouble swallowing food, but he had not felt it to be enough of a problem to mention.

> **6. If CPAP is recommended, be sure you are studied with CPAP in the sleep laboratory, so that the proper air pressure can be established to control your obstructive apnea.**

This may mean spending a second night in the laboratory. If CPAP is prescribed for you and you are simply told to "go home and try it out," find another sleep center.

Case Study. Ms. Brown had heart problems, and during an evaluation for chest pain her blood oxygen levels were checked, but sleep studies were not done. Because she snored, she was told that sleep apnea was the cause of the decrease in oxygen in her blood while sleeping. She was told to go home and use CPAP.

She slept very poorly with CPAP, but she was told to keep using it because her blood oxygen was much better.

Too frightened to stop using CPAP but exhausted from not sleeping, she was studied at an accredited sleep center. She was found to have very mild apnea, but it was central apnea, not obstructive apnea, and could not be treated effectively with CPAP.

> **7. If surgery, oral devices, medications, or weight loss are prescribed for you, be sure to have a sleep study to establish a baseline, so that it can be determined whether you are benefiting from the treatment, and if so how much.**

After treatment begins, people often feel better and think they are "cured" when, in fact, they are only partially improved. Further treatment or careful follow-up may be necessary.

Case Study. Mr. Johnson was diagnosed with severe obstructive sleep apnea. He had UPPP surgery and stopped snoring. His wife said he was cured, as she "didn't notice any more apnea." Mr. Johnson felt "much better." He was told by the surgeon that a follow-up sleep study was not necessary, since obviously he was cured.

Mr. Johnson's family doctor noticed that his blood pressure had not improved and convinced him to return to the sleep center. His follow-up sleep study showed that he had only improved 25%. On the following night he was placed on CPAP. He improved more than he could have believed, and his blood pressure dropped so far that his family doctor was able to stop one of his medications.

> **8. If you are diagnosed as having obstructive apnea but you feel that you have other reasons for feeling tired or drowsy or for having restless sleep, be sure to discuss these with your physician, because it is possible that sleep apnea may not be the most important cause of your symptoms.**

A trial with CPAP, in the sleep lab, is a good way to find out how many of your problems are caused by sleep apnea. CPAP safely eliminates any sleep apnea that you may have and you can then be the judge of whether you feel better or still have troublesome symptoms. If you are in doubt about how important sleep apnea is in causing your drowsiness, return to the laboratory for a trial with CPAP.

The opposite is also true: you may feel that you have fairly serious sleep apnea symptoms, even though your sleep test may say that your apnea is too mild for treatment. If this is the case, you may be one of those individuals who is very sensitive to sleep disruption from apnea. Discuss this possibility with your doctor. A trial with CPAP would be very helpful in letting you judge how much improvement you feel once the apnea is eliminated.

> **9. If sleep studies show that your apnea is well controlled but you continue to be sleepy, feel fatigued, or experience sleep disturbances, be sure that your doctor has considered and ruled out other conditions that might be causing those symptoms.**

As many as 20% of patients with sleep apnea have other undiagnosed sleep disorders that may not be obvious until the sleep apnea is diagnosed.

> **10. Be sure that stress factors, depression, sleep habits, and drug and alcohol use have been thoroughly discussed with you.**

Unless the physician carefully questions you about these areas, they may continue to be problems that neither you nor your doctor fully understands! Two case studies show how unexpected factors can strongly affect the results of treatment for sleep apnea.

> ***Case Study.*** *Mr. Williams was sent by his heart specialist to have a "sleep study." He was not seen by a sleep specialist but was told he had significant sleep apnea, which caused his broken sleep, chronic fatigue, headaches, and drowsiness. He was sent to have UPPP surgery, and the surgeon recommended that he go to an accredited sleep center for a reevaluation.*
>
> *The sleep specialist discovered that Mr. Williams was very depressed and had been hiding the extent of his drug and alcohol use. Mr. Williams agreed to have drug and alcohol treatment and eventually was treated with antidepressants and counseling. His sleep disorder resolved, and a sleep study showed that he had such mild apnea that further treatment was not necessary. His alcohol use and depression had aggravated his apnea and sleep-related symptoms.*

Case Study. Mr. Jones went through a divorce and became depressed. He gained a lot of weight and eventually was diagnosed as having severe sleep apnea. CPAP helped somewhat, but to the dismay of both Mr. Jones and his doctor, he had no luck losing his excess weight.

Mr. Jones was still having problems with depression, and finally went to see a psychiatrist. As counseling progressed and his depression lifted, he began to lose weight. Eventually he had UPPP surgery, his remaining mild apnea and snoring disappeared, and he was even able to discontinue CPAP.

In Mr. Jones's case neither his sleep apnea nor his weight gain was likely to improve very much until he was treated for depression.

WHAT SHOULD YOU DO IF YOU THINK YOU HAVE SLEEP APNEA?

If you think you have sleep apnea...

> **1. *First try working through your family doctor.* Make an appointment and tell him or her that you think you have sleep apnea and why you think so. Ask for a referral to an accredited sleep center to be tested for sleep apnea.**

When you see your family doctor, take with you any articles or books that have helped convince you that you have sleep apnea. You might also take along a tape recording of your snoring.

If your doctor doesn't "hear" you (that is, he is not familiar with sleep apnea or does not take your diagnosis seriously) and you are still convinced you are right...then proceed to step 2.

> **2. *Call the nearest accredited sleep center yourself.* (See the preceding section and Chap. 12.) Ask for an appointment. Some sleep centers will take patients only by referral from another physician, but many will make appointments with patients directly.**

It is always best to work with your family doctor. If you decide to contact a sleep center directly, it is still a good idea to keep your family doctor informed. For one thing he probably will become involved eventually, because the sleep clinic will probably contact him to get your medical history. Later, as a courtesy, they will probably notify him of the treatment they recommend for you. In fact, depending on the kind of treatment, your family doctor may need to become actively involved. In addition, keeping your family doctor informed will expose him to more experience with sleep apnea, which will help other people with sleep apnea in the future.

However, keep in mind that it is *your* health that is at stake, and if your doctor seems uncooperative, you should not hesitate to get in touch with a sleep center yourself.

If the closest accredited sleep center will only accept referrals and your doctor is unwilling to refer you...then take the next step.

3. Ask the sleep center for one of the following:

a. The name of a local doctor with whom they have worked who *will* refer you to the sleep clinic, or

b. The location of the closest qualified sleep center that will accept patients without a doctor's referral.

The next chapter will take you to a sleep clinic.

Summary

❖ Sleep apnea is frequently mistaken for other conditions.

❖ Misdiagnosis results in incorrect treatment, sometimes with disastrous consequences.

❖ A specialist in sleep disorders medicine at an accredited sleep center is the physician most likely to test correctly for and diagnose sleep apnea.

❖ The American Sleep Disorders Association (ASDA) can put you in touch with the nearest accredited sleep specialist or sleep center.

❖ The ten rules for avoiding misdiagnosis and the "What Should You Do...?" sections of this chapter will guide you toward an accurate diagnosis.

>>>>>>   6   >>>>>>

The Sleep Center

Testing for Sleep Apnea

THE FULL SERVICE SLEEP CENTER

Polysomnography

Sleep researchers have developed a standard way to record and measure what is going on during a person's sleep. The procedure that is used for making these recordings is called *polysomnography*, which means "making multiple sleep recordings." The electronic apparatus that is used is called (not too surprisingly) a polysomnograph.

If you have ever had an electrocardiogram (ECG or EKG) or an electroencephalogram (EEG) or if you have ever seen the way a lie detector test (polygraph) is performed, then you know exactly the kind of equipment that is used for polysomnography.

A polysomnograph records a person's sleep by gathering information from a set of little electrodes taped to the patient's skin. Wires lead from the electrodes to an electronic processor, which runs a row of pens. Each pen records the information that comes from one of the electrodes. The pens translate electrical brain signals into squiggly lines on a continuous, moving sheet of paper. The polysomnograph is able to run all night and record all the information from a full night's sleep on a very long, accordion-folded strip of paper. Many sleep centers also record and store these data by computer.

To study a person's sleep, each of the electrodes of the polysomnograph is attached with tape or a little dab of glue to a specific location on the person's skin. The electrodes are usually placed on the following places:

❖ Head, as for an EEG, to record brain wave activity that distinguishes the stages of sleep and wakefulness.

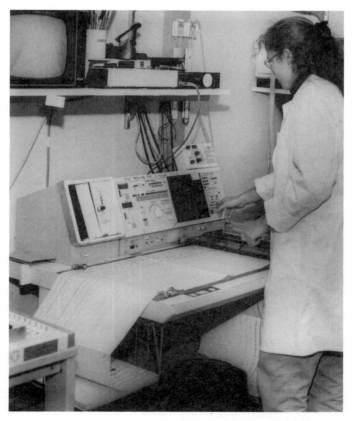

Fig. 6.1. In the control room of a sleep center, a technologist monitors a patient's sleep while it is being recorded by the polysomnograph.

✤ Face near the outside corner of each eye, to detect eye movements.

✤ Chin or throat, to detect jaw muscle tone.

✤ Chest, to pick up signals of the heartbeat, as in an ECG.

✤ Abdomen, to detect abdominal movements.

✤ Legs, to detect abnormal leg movements.

Each of these electrodes picks up information about a particular activity going on in the person's body during sleep. The recordings from each electrode can then be analyzed by comparing them with standardized "normal" recordings.

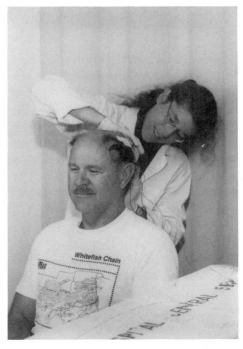

Fig. 6.2. A patient being prepared for a sleep test.

When sleep apnea is being studied, several additional recordings are made in order to gather information about the person's breathing and to show when air is moving in and out of the airway.

❖ One recording wire is attached to a stretchy belt that contains a device called a *strain gauge*. A strain gauge measures expansion, and when this belt is fastened around the person's chest, it detects expansion and contraction of the rib cage and abdomen as the muscles make breathing movements.

❖ Another recording device is an *oximeter*. It is clipped gently onto a finger or earlobe. The oximeter measures the oxygen content in the person's blood. It does this without breaking the skin, so no needles are involved.

❖ One final measurement detects air moving in and out through the nose and mouth. This is done using a small detector that rests lightly on the upper lip just beneath the nose.

Once all the electrodes and other recording devices are attached to the person being studied, the wires are gathered together into a little "pigtail," to keep them out of the way and avoid restricting freedom of movement. The bundle of wires plugs into a box, which leads to an adjacent room, where the bulk of the polysomnograph equipment is located.

It is important to emphasize that *nothing about this recording procedure hurts!* There are no needles or other pain-causing devices. The electrodes do not penetrate the skin, but are simply stuck to the surface with adhesive. And they will not cause an electrical shock.

The sleep recordings are made in a private sleep room, which is supplied with a comfortable bed. The sleep room is very well insulated, so that all outside sounds and lights are screened out, and nothing can disturb the person's sleep. The room is kept at a temperature that is comfortable for sleeping. Some sleep centers try to make the sleep rooms a little homey, with carpeting, drapes, and pictures on the walls, while other sleep rooms just look like small hospital rooms.

The Sleep Technician

Sleep technicians hook you up to the polysomnography leads, make you comfortable during the night, and monitor both your sleep and the operation of the polysomnograph equipment throughout the night. The accuracy of the results of your sleep test will depend on how carefully the technicians set you up for the test and how carefully they monitor you and the equipment. Consequently, the skill and diligence of the sleep technicians are very important.

Sleep technicians may have a wide range of training and experience, from beginners who are receiving "hands-on" training to well-trained experts who have taken courses in their field and keep up to date on the latest information on sleep testing and measurement techniques.

A sign of proficiency in this field is the credential of Registered Polysomnographic Technologist (R. Psg. T.). Sleep technicians can earn this credential by training, studying, and passing a two-day test administered by the Board of Registered Polysomnographic Technologists.

In most well-staffed sleep centers at least the supervisor of the sleep technicians will be an R. Psg. T. It is important that the person in charge of the actual sleep testing have thorough understanding of the standardized procedures for setting up and carrying out a valid sleep test. Supervision by an R. Psg. T. gives some assurance that polysomnograph equipment will be connected to the patient according to the accepted standards and that the sleep recordings will be accurate. Poorly conducted sleep tests can produce recordings that look accurate and impressive but that lead to an incorrect diagnosis.

A Visit to a Sleep Center

Let's assume that you suspect you may have sleep apnea. Your first contact with a sleep center will probably be something like Mr. Kennedy's. His wife said, "Honey, *please* do something about that snoring," so he made an initial appointment with the sleep specialist at the nearest sleep center.

Mrs. Kennedy was asked to come along with her husband to the initial discussion with the doctor. This is the usual procedure. One reason for both partners to be present is that your sleeping partner probably will be able to supply more information about your sleeping habits than you can. Another reason is that sleep disturbances like sleep apnea frequently require long-term treatment, which in some ways affects both partners. So it is a good idea for both to be part of the process from the very beginning.

At the end of Mr. Kennedy's initial interview, the sleep specialist told him he suspected sleep apnea and advised Mr. Kennedy to make an appointment for evaluation during an all-night sleep session.

Mr. Kennedy was scheduled for a date two weeks later to spend an entire night at the sleep center. He was told to plan also to spend part of the following day there for further testing. Sometimes patients spend two nights in the sleep center, but not

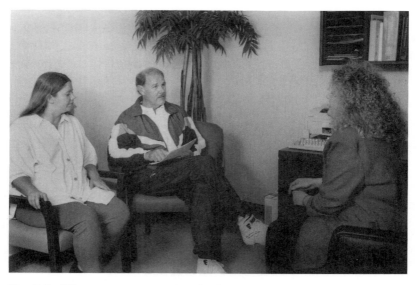

Fig. 6.3. When someone suspects he has a sleep disorder, often both he and his bedpartner will be asked to meet with the sleep specialist for the initial evaluation.

the day in between. The particular testing schedule depends on the policies and procedures of the sleep center.

On the day of Mr. Kennedy's all-night sleep session, he was asked to arrive at the sleep center in the evening, a little while before his normal bedtime, so the technician would have plenty of time to attach all the electrodes and other recording devices to him. Most sleep centers ask people to avoid alcohol, narcotics, and caffeine during the day before their sleep test, to eliminate any chance that these substances will interfere with the person's sleep.

Although he knew there was nothing painful about the procedure of recording sleep, Mr. Kennedy admits to feeling some anxiety as he arrived at the sleep center. Mr. Kennedy is not alone in having those feelings; many people are uneasy when facing an unfamiliar medical procedure.

Whenever you are undergoing any kind of medical procedure, be sure to tell the nurses or technicians if you feel nervous. They want you to be at ease. Feel free to ask questions if you are alarmed or even just curious. The technicians who prepare you for your night of sleep are so familiar with the routine that they may forget to explain the details as clearly as they should. It is okay to remind them that you are new at this and would like to understand what is going on. Everything should be clearly explained to you.

Mr. Kennedy was told he could wear his own night clothes, as long as they fit loosely and did not interfere with the placement of the electrodes. He brought a two-piece pair of pajamas, which worked fine.

When the measuring devices had all been attached and it was approximately Mr. Kennedy's normal bedtime, the technician turned out the lights and left him to go to sleep. The technician gave Mr. Kennedy a buzzer to buzz in case he needed to get up during the night to use the bathroom or needed to have the technician help him with something. Then the technician would come in and unplug his wires.

Mr. Kennedy did buzz the technician once during the night. When it seemed as though a long time had passed and the technician had not appeared, Mr. Kennedy simply unclipped the oxygen sensor from his ear. The sudden change in the signal on the polysomnograph recording told the technician that Mr. Kennedy's blood oxygen had dropped to zero. (Not a good sign!) The technician arrived instantly to reattach the sensor.

You may wonder how a person can get any sleep with so many wires attached to his body. Mr. Kennedy wondered the same thing. He was sure he would never get to sleep, but the next thing he knew the technician was telling him it was morning. Despite the unusual setting, most people manage to get a fairly decent night's sleep.

The reason Mr. Kennedy was asked to stay for part of the next day was for something called a *multiple sleep latency test* (MSLT). *Sleep latency* is a measure of how long it takes a person to fall asleep during the daytime. It indicates the degree of excessive daytime sleepiness that the person is experiencing. As you already know, excessive daytime sleepiness is one of the symptoms of sleep apnea.

To measure sleep latency, Mr. Kennedy was simply asked to return to his sleep room several times during the day for

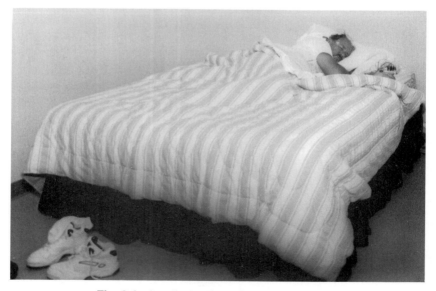

Fig. 6.4. A patient asleep during a sleep test.

20-minute rest periods. He would lie down for 20 minutes while the polysomnograph recorded whether he fell asleep and exactly how long it took to do so.

In between MSLT naps you will be unplugged from the recorder and will be free to walk around, read, watch television, or even go to the cafeteria for lunch. Of course, you will still have all your electrodes attached and a clump of wires dangling around your neck. Some people are not bothered a bit by this. Others, like Mr. Kennedy, feel a little like Frankenstein's monster and prefer to have lunch delivered so they do not have to wander very far from the sleep center.

If you are staying in the sleep center for an MSLT, be sure to bring along something to entertain yourself: a book or magazine, crossword puzzles, needlework, a deck of cards. If you object to

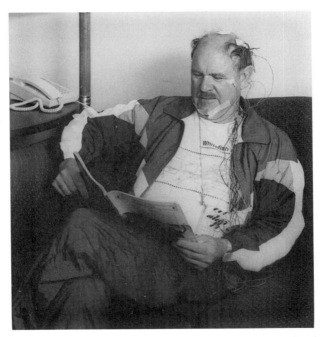

Fig. 6.5. A patient killing time in the sleep center during the day, between MSLTs.

wandering around in your bathrobe all day, you might bring some loose-fitting day-wear, such as a caftan or a jogging suit, which can be worn comfortably over the wires.

After all the recordings are completed, the doctor will read through the graph-paper records of your sleep night, looking for signs that tell him whether you have sleep apnea, and, if so, what kind and how severe it is. Another appointment will be scheduled for you to discuss the results and, if necessary, talk with you about treatment.

AT-HOME SLEEP TESTING: PORTABLE MONITORING

A recent trend is toward at-home testing, also called *portable monitoring* or *ambulatory monitoring*. As a means of testing for sleep disorders, this technology is still under development. In the spring of 1993 the American Sleep Disorders Association (ASDA) issued its first set of recommendations on the standards and practices for portable sleep testing. If professional standards can be established, at-home monitoring may allow less expensive diagnostic or follow-up testing *for some selected patients* and may free the sleep labs to treat a larger volume of patients.

At-home testing can be carried out in several ways. One alternative is for the patient to come to the sleep lab in the evening, have the monitoring equipment hooked up to him, and then wear it home and sleep with it. Another method is for a technologist to come to the patient's home to set up the equipment. The technologist might be either someone from the sleep center or a specially trained representative from a homecare or medical equipment company.

At present, several questions and problems remain to be solved with regard to sleep testing by ambulatory monitoring. One important question is, "For which patients—and for which sleep disorders—is this technique appropriate?" For people suspected of having obstructive sleep apnea, the ASDA considers at-home testing appropriate if the symptoms are obvious and severe and if the person urgently needs treatment but cannot easily get to a sleep lab for a standard test.

On the other hand, certain people may not be good candidates for ambulatory monitoring. For people with very mild symptoms some of the simpler versions of at-home testing may not produce enough data for a good diagnosis. For people suspected of having narcolepsy, ambulatory monitoring may be insufficient because an MSLT is usually needed for the diagnosis.

A sleep test performed at home must be as thorough as a test performed in the sleep center. If an at-home sleep study is suggested to you, ask whether the same number of measurements will be recorded as in a sleep center study. Do not accept assurances lightly; make sure that the test will actually monitor your *sleep.* This means that sensors should be attached to your head to monitor brain waves (EEG), eye movements (EOG), and chin movements (EMG) and that other sensors should be attached for heart rate, breathing or airflow, oxygen saturation, and body movements. Many different portable monitoring arrangements exist, each collecting data by means of a variety of sensors in varying numbers and combinations. For example, eight "leads" attached to the body will collect less data than 12. Some monitoring arrangements fail to detect arousals; some do not record breathing or leg movements. For very sick people with serious heart or breathing problems and for patients who require an extremely accurate measurement of sleep stages or of "sleepiness" (EDS), ambulatory monitoring may not produce a precise enough record to be acceptable.

Another issue is the training and skill of the medical staff carrying out the test. A test set up by a poorly trained technician or analyzed by an unqualified person can generate misleading results. The ASDA standards specify that only a licensed physician may order a portable sleep test and that the individuals who set up and evaluate the test should be certified or eligible for certification.

Finally, there is the question of cost-effectiveness for the patient and/or his insurance company. At-home testing promises to be cheaper than in-lab testing. However, in how many instances will at-home tests need to be followed up and verified by in-lab tests?

Some proponents of ambulatory monitoring claim that people's sleep is more "normal" during an at-home test than in the sleep lab. However, there is no clear evidence to prove this, nor to prove that at-home testing is necessarily more comfortable for the patient. For some people an at-home test may have numerous drawbacks. Sleep may be disturbed by other family members, by the home surroundings, by neighborhood noises, and by other interruptions that are not present in a sleep center. Further, if sensors become disconnected during the night, no attendant is present to replace them and make sure that the sleep study is complete.

Ambulatory monitoring has some strong advocates. Among these are some small sleep labs that are not equipped to test large numbers of patients. For these labs the ability to test patients at home is an advantage.

Homecare and equipment manufacturers are also interested in expanding into the business of at-home testing. They would supply the equipment, send a technician to the patient's home to set up the test, and send the results to a physician for analysis. The ASDA recommends against any arrangement in which the company conducting the test stands to profit from the results by selling the patient a CPAP unit or homecare services. The possibility for conflict of interest here is obvious.

Unless and until professional standards such as those recommended by the ASDA are agreed upon and followed, at-home testing can be expected to vary widely in its accuracy and cost-effectiveness.

DETERMINING THE SEVERITY OF SLEEP APNEA

When is a person's sleep apnea severe enough to cause concern? Sleep specialists define "clinical" sleep apnea (sleep apnea that needs medical attention) in the following terms:

❖ An *apnea event* is when breathing stops for *more than ten seconds.*

❖ A person is considered to have "clinical" sleep apnea if he has *more than five apnea events per hour.*

This definition determines whether the person has sleep apnea, but it tells only part of the story.

The next question is, "How severe is the sleep apnea?" How sick is this person? The sleep specialist needs to answer this question to decide on the appropriate treatment.

Sleep specialists use several "yardsticks" to determine the severity of a person's sleep apnea. The simplest measure, now somewhat outdated, is called the *apnea index*. This is just the number of apnea events per hour of sleep: a person who has 30 apnea events per hour of sleep would have an apnea index of 30.

Another measurement is the total number of apnea events during an entire night. As an example, 250 apneas in an eight-hour night would not be unusual for a person with moderately serious sleep apnea.

A more accurate measure than the apnea index is the *Apnea-plus-Hypopnea Index (AHI)*, also called the *Respiratory Disturbance Index (RDI)*. (Hypopnea is abnormally shallow breathing. A *hypopnea event* is a partially obstructed breath and is characteristic of sleep apnea.) The AHI (or RDI) expresses the total number of apneas plus hypopneas. The combined totals are a more refined measure of the severity of sleep apnea than a simple count of apnea events alone.

Even the RDI may not give the full picture of sleep apnea severity. Another important indicator is *oxygen saturation*—the amount of oxygen present in the blood. Some people, despite a fairly small number of apnea events, may still be quite sick because of a very low oxygen saturation. So the measure of oxygen saturation is an important part of the total sleep apnea picture. Oxygen saturation is measured as a percentage. Normal is about 95%, and decreases slightly as we get older. In people with sleep apnea a blood oxygen content of 80% or so during sleep is fairly common. Levels below 70% are considered critically low, because of the high probability of irregular heart rhythm at lower blood oxygen levels.

A further aspect of the severity of sleep apnea and the need for treatment is the question of daytime sleepiness: is sleepiness interfering with the person's life? Some people are more sensitive to sleepiness than others, and alertness is more critical for some than for others (for example, an airplane pilot or a school bus driver). The results of the multiple sleep latency test (MSLT), described earlier, give a good measurement of a person's tendency to fall asleep during the day.

DECIDING WHO NEEDS TREATMENT

After your sleep test, in a follow-up visit or phone call, your sleep specialist will review with you your sleep test results: RDI, oxygen saturation record, the results of your MSLT. These data and consideration of your overall health will help him decide whether your sleep apnea is serious enough to need treatment.

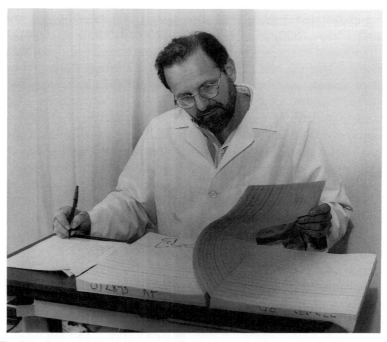

Fig. 6.6. A trained sleep center staff member studies and "scores" the results of a polysomnograph test. The score indicates the kind of sleep disorder and its severity. The paper on this table is the result of one patient's sleep test.

People usually need immediate treatment if their excessive drowsiness interferes with such daily activities as driving, if it creates job hazards, if they have heart failure related to sleep apnea, or if they have very low oxygen saturation during the night. People who feel constantly tired or who have worsening high blood pressure, heart arrhythmias related to sleep apnea, badly disrupted sleep, or an AHI of more than 40 also usually need treatment.

If a person's symptoms are less severe or the results of the sleep study show mild sleep apnea, the sleep specialist will have to consider carefully the whole picture before deciding whether to recommend treatment and, if so, how aggressive the treatment should be. See Chapter 7 for treatment of sleep apnea.

Summary

❖ *Sleep testing involves sleeping for a night at a sleep center while a device called a polysomnograph electronically records your sleep.*

❖ *You may also be asked to spend part of the next day at the sleep center for a Multiple Sleep Latency Test (MSLT).*

❖ *From the results of these tests, the sleep specialist will*

    Decide whether you have sleep apnea; and, if so,

    Determine how severe it is; and

    Rule out other disorders that might accompany the sleep apnea.

>>>>> 7 >>>>>

Treating Sleep Apnea

*M*r. Kennedy had a complete sleep test at an accredited sleep center. The test results showed that he had more than 250 apnea events during the night while his sleep was being recorded. He was judged to be suffering from moderately severe obstructive sleep apnea with a minor central apnea component, and he had cardiac arrhythmia. His sleep specialist recommended that he undergo treatment.

At this point, Mr. Kennedy had answers to the first two questions on the pathway to successful treatment of sleep apnea:

1. Is his condition actually sleep apnea, and does he have any other conditions that will have a bearing on successful treatment?

2. What kind of sleep apnea is it (central, obstructive, or mixed) and how severe is it? (The answer to this question is important because it determines the kind of treatment.)

Finally comes the third and crucial question:

3. What is the most conservative treatment for Mr. Kennedy's type of sleep apnea that has a good chance of success?

CHOOSING THE MOST CONSERVATIVE TREATMENT

The choice of treatment should be explored carefully by you, your sleep specialist, and perhaps your family doctor, once a diagnosis has been made. What is the most conservative treatment for you? This is a complex and individual question that needs to be answered on the basis of the kind of apnea you have, how severe it is, and your overall health. Your sleep specialist can describe the various treatments that may be effective for you and can tell you which ones are the most conservative.

What do we mean by *most conservative*? This means the treatment that carries the *lowest risk for you.*

Keep in mind that different doctors may have different treatment recommendations. Every doctor has conscious and unconscious biases in favor of certain forms of treatment. This is a natural result of a doctor's training and specialization. For example, a surgeon is more likely than an internist to believe that surgery is the best option; an internist might lean toward a nonsurgical treatment.

Your job is to take these possible biases into account as you and your doctors weigh the risks and benefits and choose the most appropriate treatment for you. Some treatment options involve surgery. Before deciding on surgery it is always wise to get a second opinion from a different physician.

The most conservative treatments for sleep apnea do not involve surgery. They may involve some inconvenience or perseverance; but they do not expose the patient to the risks of pain and suffering and possible complications or death that are inherent in any surgical procedure.

After the nonsurgical options, the next most conservative treatments are the simplest surgical procedures. A surgical procedure could be considered "simple" if it meets most or all of the following criteria:

❖ It is a routine procedure that has been carried out for many years, rather than a new or experimental type of surgery.

✤ It does not involve cutting major blood vessels or nerves, dealing with major organs, or entering a body cavity.

✤ It normally has no serious postoperative complications.

✤ It can be done by a surgeon who is experienced with this particular surgical procedure.

✤ It can be done on an outpatient basis or involves, at most, a minimal (one- or two-day) hospital stay.

Surgery has many pitfalls: pain, excessive loss of blood, reactions to medications, nerve or muscle damage, infection, wound breakdown, and other complications.[1,2]

One of the biggest risks from surgery is general anesthesia.[1] This is particularly true for a person with sleep apnea. Anesthetics depress the breathing reflexes, and a person with sleep apnea already has some degree of respiratory difficulty. Anyone with sleep apnea who is having surgery should warn his surgeon in advance that he has sleep apnea. Better yet, he could ask his sleep specialist to consult with the surgeon. The surgeon and the anesthesiologist should *both* be aware that this person's breathing will need to be monitored very carefully during and immediately after surgery.

So even "simple" surgery should be considered very carefully. For a person who is very sick as a result of sleep apnea, surgery may be the only option that makes sense: it may be necessary to save his life. For other people who are not in immediate danger from the severe long-term effects of apnea or who may simply want to "stop snoring," the potential risks involved in surgery may outweigh the possible benefits.

It is extremely important to realize that the reconstructive surgical procedures for sleep apnea are not equally effective for all people. For example, the most "popular" surgical procedure for sleep apnea, UPPP, described later, has about a 50% failure rate, and after five years the success rate may fall to as low as 25%. This means that half the people who undergo this surgery still have a significant problem with sleep apnea immediately after surgery, and the percentage of people with problems continues to increase with time.

Surgery for reconstructing the lower jaw (mandibular advancement and its variations) also has a fairly high nonsuccess rate.

There are several reasons for the failure of surgery to correct sleep apnea. One is simply inappropriate choice of treatment. There are some patients for whom it can be predicted in advance that UPPP is not likely to cure their apnea. Yet some of these patients choose to have surgery anyway. Quite often, after a person is told he has sleep apnea, he is not ready to think of himself as having a long-term health condition. He may seize upon surgery as a hopeful "quick fix." Or the person may be referred directly to a surgeon by a family doctor who is unfamiliar with recent advances in nonsurgical treatments for sleep apnea. Poor surgical candidates usually find that their sleep apnea returns after surgery and that they still need long-term treatment.

Another reason for the high percentage of unsuccessful surgery is the newness of treating sleep apnea with surgery: there still are not enough data to be able to predict accurately which people will be cured by a particular reconstructive procedure.

So before you choose surgery for the treatment of sleep apnea, ask your doctor about the chances of success for you, and *listen carefully to his answer.*

To summarize, it makes sense to be sure you are an *excellent* candidate for the particular kind of surgery you are considering, before you take the risk of having it. A second opinion from a qualified sleep specialist or an internist familiar with sleep apnea is strongly advised.

One final point on choosing a conservative treatment: if you are considering being treated at a medical school, you might keep in mind that medical schools may lean toward more aggressive, more experimental, less conservative treatment options. Although this is fine from the point of view of advancing medical science, ask yourself whether you want to risk becoming part of that process.

WHO TREATS SLEEP APNEA?

Where your treatment will be carried out will depend both on your sleep center and on the treatment you will have. Some sleep centers provide both testing and treatment of sleep apnea, many do only sleep testing, and some fall in between these two extremes, doing some types of treatment in-house but referring patients elsewhere for others.

In any case, you can expect the sleep specialist and his staff to work with you and your family to plan your treatment and to recommend a treatment specialist. Your family doctor may be brought into the process at this stage.

Your sleep doctor may begin by suggesting a number of treatments that you can carry out on your own (stop smoking, lose weight, and so on). To help you with these the sleep center may refer you to a nutritional counselor, a smokers' support group, or other such organized programs.

If surgery is an option for you and your sleep center does not perform surgery, the center will probably suggest or recommend surgeons and other specialists with whom its staff members work frequently, and these physicians will be brought into the picture to help plan your treatment.

If your sleep center has surgeons and other specialists on the staff who can treat you right there, you may still want to talk with an outside physician, preferably one with some familiarity with sleep disorders, for a second opinion before you agree to surgery.

If your treatment involves medications, the sleep center may prefer to start you off on the medication and then have your family physician take over the follow-up care and keep an eye on your progress.

The most common treatment involves the use of a breathing device. The device may be supplied through the sleep center, or

they may arrange for a homecare or medical equipment company to supply the equipment.

So, you see, how you receive your treatment will depend on
the particular sleep center, the size of its staff, and the emphasis
of its program. (See Chaps. 13 and 14 for more on how to obtain
the health care services you need.)

THE FIRST STEP IN TREATMENT: ELIMINATE THE OBVIOUS

The first step in treating sleep apnea is to eliminate anything
that is aggravating your problem. This may improve your sleep
apnea symptoms enough that you can avoid more complicated
forms of treatment. The following can all increase symptoms:

❖ *Alcohol*, especially in the evening (even a single glass of
   wine with dinner), can increase the number of apnea events
   and decrease the oxygen in the blood during the night. A
   person with sleep apnea should avoid alcohol in the
   evening.

❖ *Smoking* decreases the amount of oxygen in the blood and
   causes swelling of the lining of the airway, which contributes
   to obstructive apnea. People with sleep apnea would be prudent to stop smoking.

❖ *Allergies* and *respiratory infections* also cause swelling and
   obstruction of the airway. Treatment of allergies and upper
   airway infections can diminish the symptoms of obstructive
   sleep apnea.

❖ *Evening medications,* such as tranquilizers and short-acting
   beta blockers, can sometimes worsen sleep apnea. The
   sleep specialist may want to consult with the physician who
   prescribed the medication to see whether a change in prescription or in medication schedule can help eliminate

sleep apnea symptoms. (See Appendix for list of medications that affect sleep.)

✤ *Obesity* contributes greatly to obstructive sleep apnea, and weight loss can be helpful. Weight loss is discussed in detail later in the section on treating obstructive sleep apnea and in Chapter 8.

Some of these aggravating factors involve habits that are difficult for people to change or give up. Often people have the best results if they are enrolled in an organized program to help them eliminate the habit. If you find yourself trying to deal with a stubborn problem such as losing weight or stopping smoking, ask your sleep center to recommend a program that has been helpful to other people.

TREATMENTS FOR CENTRAL APNEA

Drugs

Drugs that stimulate the breathing reflexes are, at present, the most common treatments for central apnea. Unfortunately, most of the drugs have drawbacks that make them less than ideal. Some are not very effective; some work for a while but the person may develop a tolerance to the drug; and some have undesirable side effects. Consequently, the drugs available today for treating central apnea should be considered temporary measures, and we must hope that research in this field will soon offer more acceptable alternatives.

Acetazolamide is the drug that has received the most attention. It makes the blood more acidic, which tends to stimulate the breathing reflex. Experiments have shown that acetazolamide can decrease the number of apnea events and result in a modest decrease in daytime sleepiness.[3] However, other studies are less enthusiastic,[4] and there are reports of this drug leading to the development of obstructive apnea.[5] More research is needed, but at present acetazolamide is the most promising drug for treatment of central apnea.

Another drug that has provided some improvement in central apnea is *clomipramine*, an antidepressant. It has been used on only a few patients and has resulted in improved sleep and respiration and fewer apnea events. However, some patients developed a tolerance to the drug after six to 12 months, after which it was no longer effective. In addition, clomipramine has some undesirable side effects, one of which is impotence.[6,7]

A third drug that has been tried experimentally on central apnea with some encouraging results is *doxapram*.[6] This is a respiratory stimulant that is normally used only for the short term (one or two hours at a time) to stimulate the breathing of patients who are recovering from anesthesia. It has never been recommended for long-term use, and it has some serious side effects, including hyperactivity, irregular heart rhythms, increased blood pressure, nausea and diarrhea, and urinary retention. It should not be used in people with heart disease, high blood pressure, and perhaps heart rhythm irregularities. These categories include many of the people who have serious complications from sleep apnea. It remains to be seen how useful this drug will be.

Other drugs that have been tried, with very little improvement in the central apnea, are *aminophylline* and *theophylline*, bronchodilators normally used to treat asthma and emphysema; *almitrine*, a breathing stimulant; *naloxone*, a drug that has been used to counteract the depression of the breathing reflexes that results from morphine, codeine, and so on; *medroxyprogesterone*, a hormone similar to the female hormone progesterone, which is known to stimulate respiration; and *tryptophan*, an amino acid that reportedly acts as an antidepressant. None of these has had dramatic effects on central apnea. All of them except tryptophan have serious undesirable side effects.[6–12]

Oxygen has also been tried, with mixed results.[13]

With so many drugs in existence and being developed each year, one hopes that drugs will soon be found that provide specific treatment for people with central apnea without serious side effects. Much more vigorous research in this field is needed.

Breathing Devices

Diaphragmatic Pacemaker

A diaphragmatic pacemaker works very much like a heart pacemaker: it uses tiny, rhythmic pulses of electric current to stimulate rhythmic muscle contractions. Diaphragmatic pacemakers were first developed to treat victims of polio whose breathing reflexes no longer operated. However, the devices were never used much for this purpose because "iron lungs" were developed and because the availability of polio vaccine soon eliminated the need.

Since then some work has been done using diaphragmatic pacemakers in patients with spinal cord injuries, whose breathing reflexes have been interrupted, and in infants born with faulty breathing reflexes. And a few diaphragmatic pacemakers have been tried on adult patients with central sleep apnea.

In theory this seems like an ideal solution. Central apnea is essentially the absence of the nerve signal that goes to the diaphragm during sleep to tell it to breathe. A pacemaker, used during sleep, should be able to supply that signal. However, this technology has not advanced very rapidly, and the diaphragmatic pacemaker has not yet become widely available, probably partly because until recently the demand was not there. With better recognition of central sleep apnea, demand may increase.

Implanting the pacemaker requires delicate surgery, to place a pair of tiny electrodes next to the phrenic nerves (the nerves that control the diaphragm). This is done either in the neck, using a local anesthetic, or in the chest cavity, using general anesthesia. Usually both nerves, one on each side of the body, are used rather than just one, which would only stimulate one side of the diaphragm. During surgery, a small receiver also is placed underneath the skin.[14,15] To use the pacemaker, a radio frequency generator is placed against the skin over the implanted receiver, and radio frequency pulses stimulate the phrenic nerve.

Some problems and risks are involved in using a diaphragmatic pacemaker on a person with sleep apnea. One drawback is that it can cause obstructive apnea to emerge, which raises a whole new set of issues.[16] However, the most serious risk is the possibility of damaging the phrenic nerve, either during surgery or at some later time. Loss of both phrenic nerves, of course, would leave the person with a paralyzed diaphragm and unable to breathe well on his own. For this reason the operation must be done with meticulous care to avoid the slightest damage to the nerves.

Should you be considering this type of surgery, you would be wise to go to whatever lengths are necessary to locate a medical center that has an extensive history of installing and using diaphragmatic pacemakers and to find the surgeon who is most experienced with the procedure.

At present a diaphragmatic pacemaker probably is not a practical treatment option for most people with central apnea, although it can be considered for some patients. As research is done and experience is gained, these devices may become a more attractive method of treatment.

Mechanical Ventilators

Several forms of mechanical breathing systems can be used to assist breathing during sleep by people with central apnea. These devices operate either by "positive pressure" (forcing air into the lungs in a rhythmic, breathing-like pattern) or by "negative pressure" (more or less mimicking the actions of the breathing muscles).

Positive pressure ventilators operate by rhythmically pushing air into the airway through a tube. Usually the air tube enters the body by way of a tracheostomy, a direct opening in the throat (described later). However, in emergencies or in very sick people the tube may be inserted through the nose or mouth, or the person may be ventilated with a face mask or nasal mask.

A positive-pressure ventilator is less cumbersome than a negative-pressure ventilator, and its use is becoming more common as better ventilators and face masks become available.

A negative-pressure ventilator works differently. The best-known example of a negative-pressure ventilator is probably the "iron lung," developed in the 1930s to "breathe" for polio victims who had lost their breathing reflexes. An iron lung works by rhythmically lowering the air pressure in a chamber surrounding the person's body. When the pressure around the body drops, the lungs expand and air flows into them. Your diaphragm normally operates in exactly this way: by contracting downward it lowers the pressure inside your rigid chest cavity and allows your lungs to expand and fill with air.

A number of miniaturized versions of the iron lung have been developed that surround only the chest. One such system is called a cuirass, named for the rigid piece of armor that was worn over the upper body by medieval knights. The ventilator cuirass fits closely over the chest of the person lying in bed. The cuirass is connected to an air pump, which rhythmically lowers the pressure between the cuirass and the chest, enabling air to enter the lungs. For the cuirass to work effectively, the seal between the shield and the body must be very good. Some people have difficulty getting a good fit.

Mechanical ventilators have had their problems. The rhythm can be tricky to adjust; it must be regulated to breathe at the proper rate for the person using it. A mechanical system that completely controls breathing is uncomfortable for people who are somewhat able to breathe on their own and need only occasional assistance. The newest generation of ventilators minimizes this discomfort by allowing the person to breathe on his own as much as he can and to assist breathing only if he stops.

Though cumbersome, these breathing systems can be effective for many people who have central apnea and are unable to sleep and breathe at the same time.

CPAP

CPAP (continuous positive airway pressure) is a breathing system that has been used successfully to treat obstructive sleep apnea. It was devised in 1981 by Sullivan and his group at the University of Sydney Medical School in Australia.[17]

A few patients with central apnea have been tried on CPAP with some success.[18] Some patients who appear to have central sleep apnea may improve on nasal bi-pressure therapy (BiPAP). Others will have little if any improvement. Treatment of central apnea is still being investigated. (For more information about CPAP and BiPAP, see the later section on treating obstructive sleep apnea.)

The choice of treatment for central apnea should be made only after a thorough consultation with your sleep specialist.

TREATMENTS FOR OBSTRUCTIVE AND MIXED APNEAS

Obstructive and mixed apnea are easier to treat than central apnea. The current methods of treating obstructive sleep apnea are (from most conservative to least) change of sleeping position, weight loss, breathing devices, oral devices, drugs, and surgery.

Mixed apnea generally is treated by first treating the obstructive apnea component. Once the obstructive apnea is under control, the central apnea almost always ceases to be a problem.

Change of Sleep Position

People with obstructive sleep apnea generally have more severe apnea events when sleeping on their backs; a few people have breathing difficulties *only* while lying on their backs. For these few people a change in sleep position may eliminate the problem. However, there is no good evidence that this technique produces reliable results each night.

Some individuals' apnea is so severe that even brief periods of apnea are life-threatening, and position training is not helpful.

The people most likely to be helped by position change are those

1. Whose obstructive apnea has been shown during a sleep study to occur only while lying on their back; and

2. Who can reliably sleep on their side.

Learning to avoid a particular sleep position is a matter of conditioning. Several sleep position monitors and alarms have been developed that alert the sleeper when he rolls onto his back and train him to choose a different sleep position. A simple method to try is to sew a small ball into the back of the pajamas. (See the Appendix.) A couple of weeks of practice may be needed before a new sleep position becomes a habit, and a person may need to "retrain" himself periodically.

Weight Loss

Who Can Be Helped by Weight Loss?

This treatment option can be effective for people with the Pickwickian syndrome (see Chap. 8) and many other overweight heavy snorers

1. Whose apnea is associated primarily with their weight gain rather than with an anatomic obstruction of the airway (tonsils, uvula, tongue); and

2. Whose life is not in immediate danger from the effects of sleep apnea, such as sleepiness or heart disease.[19–21]

The people who are most likely to be successful at weight loss are overweight apnea sufferers who are highly motivated to improve their health and lifestyle.

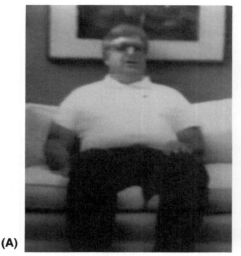 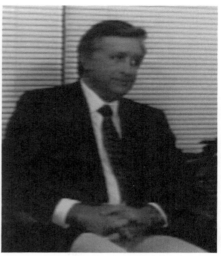

(A)   **(B)**

FIG. 7.1. A successful weight loss patient, **(A)** before treatment for sleep apnea, and **(B)** five years later.

Why Does Weight Loss Work?

Weight loss, when it is effective, works for two reasons: it relieves the abnormal loading upon the abdomen that interferes, in some cases, with breathing reflexes; and it reduces the fatty deposits in the throat tissue that contribute to the development of obstructive apnea. However, weight loss is only effective if

1. Sufficient weight is lost; and

2. The weight can be kept off permanently.

Insufficient weight loss and weight regained are the two main reasons for this treatment failing, when it does fail. In fact, there may be a kind of weight "threshold," above which extra weight causes apnea symptoms and below which the symptoms are relieved.[19] According to this theory, you will need to reduce your weight far enough to fall below that threshold before you can expect to see significant improvement in your apnea symptoms.

Losing weight and keeping it off may be difficult or impossible for some people as long as their sleep apnea is untreated. Their fatigue, sleepiness, low energy, and reduced vigor may prevent them from being physically active enough to burn calories, build muscle, and successfully lose weight. In these cases the combination of CPAP (discussed later) and weight loss can have dramatic results (see Fig. 7.1). (For more on obesity, sleep apnea, and weight loss, see Chap. 8.)

Weight loss surgery is a radical way of losing weight. It is not a conservative treatment, and is discussed later in the section on surgery.

CPAP and Similar Breathing Devices

Breathing devices that treat obstructive apnea do so by using air pressure as a "splint" to hold the upper airway open and keep it from collapsing during sleep. Some sleep experts believe that, in addition, the higher-than-normal air pressure delivered by these devices may stimulate the person's breathing reflexes. However, the primary role of air pressure devices is to act as an airway splint.

The most commonly used version of this system is called **CPAP** (Continuous Positive Airway Pressure). As mentioned earlier, CPAP (pronounced "SEE-pap") was developed as a treatment for sleep apnea by Sullivan and his research group in Australia in 1981.[17] It was first used to treat sleep apnea patients in the United States in 1984.

CPAP is extremely effective. In fact, it is the most effective nonsurgical treatment for obstructive sleep apnea. For that reason CPAP has become the treatment of choice at most sleep centers.

The standard CPAP system consists of a small, soft, rubbery mask worn over the nose (not the mouth) at night. The mask is connected by flexible tubing to an air pump, which provides continuous air pressure through the tubing and into the nose (Figs. 7.2 and 7.3). As soon as the CPAP wearer begins to inhale, the air pressure stabilizes his soft palate and tongue and prevents his airway from collapsing. A pressure regulator is

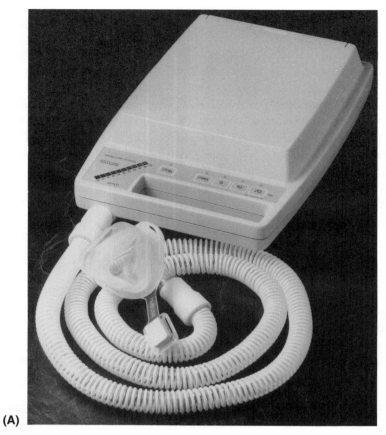

(A)

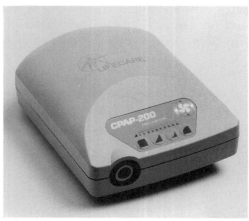

(B)

FIG. 7.2. Examples of CPAP units. **(A)** Res-Care Sullivan® APD-2s CPAP system shown with Bubble Mask™. **(B)** Lifecare CPAP–200™

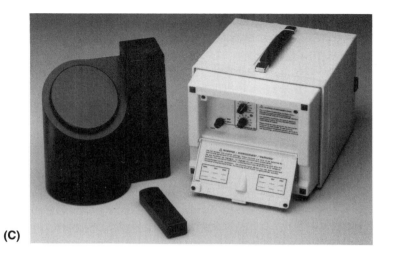

(C)

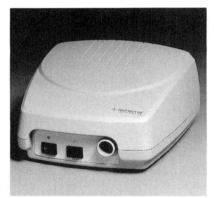

(D)

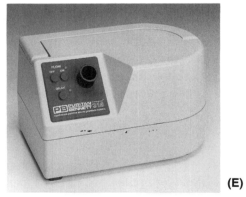

(E)

FIG. 7.2. Continued. **(C)** Respironics REMstar Choice® CPAP system (*left*), with remote control, and Respironics BiPAP® system (*right*). **(D)** Healthdyne Quest™ CPAP system. **(E)** Puritan-Bennett Companion® 318 CPAP system.

custom-set for him during a night in the sleep lab, so that the CPAP delivers exactly enough air pressure to prevent his apnea events, but no higher than necessary.

CPAP pressure is measured in centimeters of water (cm H_2O), in much the same way that barometric pressure is measured in millimeters of mercury (mm Hg). Typical CPAP pressure settings range from 5 to 20 cm H_2O.

Who Can Benefit from Using CPAP?

CPAP can produce a virtual "miracle" cure in people who have not slept and breathed normally in years and are extremely ill from the cardiac and respiratory effects of years of sleep apnea. There are probably more than 200,000 people in the United States using CPAP today, with the numbers growing by the tens of thousands each year. However, many people have trouble adapting to the use of CPAP.

Treatment with CPAP should always be started and evaluated in the sleep center during an overnight sleep study. This allows the sleep technician to adjust the pressure correctly, establish a baseline for monitoring the effectiveness of the treatment, and avoid inappropriate or ineffectual use of CPAP.

Getting Used to CPAP

The use of CPAP requires some motivation and perseverance. A few minutes are needed before going to bed each night, to wash the face so the skin is clean and will not be irritated by the mask, and a few more minutes every morning to wash the mask. In addition, one simply needs to make a commitment to use the system each night for reasons of better health and longer life. (See Chaps. 14 and 15 for more on using CPAP.)

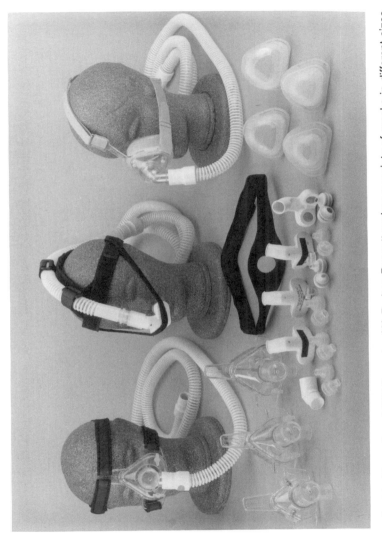

FIG. 7.3. Examples of CPAP masks. **(A)** Puritan-Bennett makes a variety of masks in different sizes, and also The Adam device (nasal "pillows").

(A)

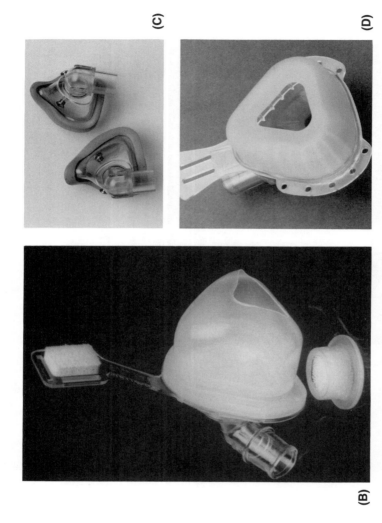

FIG. 7.3. Continued. **(B)** ResCare Bubble Mask™, showing thin, single-layer cushion. In front, a ResCare disposable Hygroscopic Condenser Humidifier (HCH). **(C)** Lifecare Softwear® Nasal Mask, shown in two sizes. **(D)** Healthdyne Soft Series.

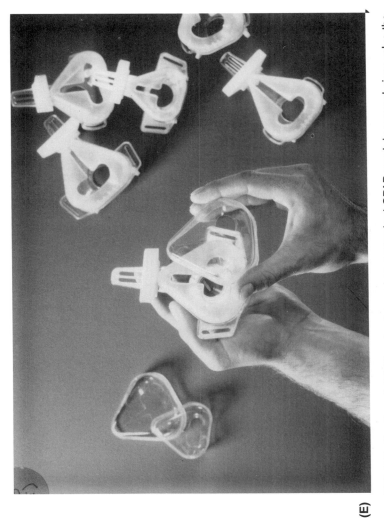

FIG. 7.3. Continued. **(E)** Respironics makes a standard CPAP mask in several sizes, plus the Comfort Flap™ featuring a thin, replaceable cover.

(E)

95

CPAP users generally are willing to put up with the inconvenience of CPAP once they experience the results. In one follow-up study of 20 CPAP users after about a year, 16 were still using their CPAP all night, every night.[22] Such a high degree of compliance with the treatment reflects the users' enthusiasm about its effectiveness.

The main drawbacks with CPAP are related to its clumsiness and its effect on sleep and to its tendency to cause nasal irritation in some people. Some people can get used to wearing the mask in just one or two nights; others may take several weeks. The air pump motor makes a fanlike sound that a few CPAP user find to be too loud, but most do not object to it; their bedpartners generally find CPAP much easier to sleep with than explosive snoring. (See Chap. 15 for ideas on how to cut down on CPAP sound.)

The mask tends to restrict movement a little during sleep, because the easiest position for sleeping while wearing the mask is on the back. It is possible to turn from side to side, but a little care has to be taken not to dislodge the mask. The flexible Bubble Mask™ and the nasal "pillows" have eliminated a lot of this problem.

The blower unit that generates the air pressure can also be clumsy to live with. Some units are about the size of an automobile battery and weigh about 10 pounds; others are small enough to fit into a briefcase and weigh as little as 4.5 pounds. People who are dedicated to using CPAP don't like to sleep without it, and they carry their units on business trips and vacations, but not without some inconvenience. The manufacturers of CPAP systems are continually working on refinements, and their newer models are becoming ever smaller and less cumbersome. Today's CPAPs will fit easily under an airplane seat. Some come with their own carrying case. (See Chap. 13 on choosing a CPAP.)

CPAP causes nasal congestion and sneezing in some people. This can often be helped by using a humidifier. (See Chap. 15 for CPAP problem-solving tips.)

Some people simply refuse to wear the CPAP mask because it gives them a sense of claustrophobia or for other reasons. The staff of the sleep center and the homecare company that supplies the CPAP should be able to help most people solve their CPAP adjustment problems. (An alternative to the standard mask is discussed later. See also Chaps. 14 and 15.)

People who use CPAP regularly occasionally stop using it for a while. But they generally return to it quickly because their apnea symptoms promptly return. In fact, after using CPAP and then sleeping without it, one person reported that he had never been so aware of the choking he experienced with each apnea event. Before he used CPAP, he was not even aware that he was struggling for air all night long. Now if he sleeps without CPAP, he dreams that heavy weights have been placed on his chest, or he awakens feeling suffocated. So he is not often tempted to give up his CPAP.

CPAP provides positive results that are close to an instant cure. After beginning to use CPAP, most people report that within days they feel better than they have felt in many years. They report sleeping better, feeling rested in the morning and alert during the day, and having the energy to do the things they have been longing to do.

What Are the Long-Term Effects of Using CPAP?

CPAP is a relatively recent development, having only been in use in the United States since about 1985. Sleep researchers have been watching carefully for any unfavorable long-term effects. By now hundreds of people have been using CPAP for more than seven years, and no serious negative consequences have been reported in the medical literature. Of course, no one can guarantee the safety of sleeping for ten or 20 years under slightly higher air pressure. But so far the medical literature suggests that the long-term risks from sleep apnea are much more dangerous than the possibility of long-term risks from using CPAP.

How Much Do CPAP Devices Cost?

CPAP systems can be obtained by rental or purchase. It is a good idea to begin by renting a system for two or three months and seeing how you do with it. Costs vary around the country. At this writing, CPAP rentals are approximately $200 per month, and the purchase price is in the neighborhood of $1,200. You may have to purchase the mask and tubing separately (about $130). The mask material tends to absorb oil from the skin and become stiff, so masks require periodic replacement (about $50). Older masks lasted only about six months; newer, silicone ones may last up to 18 months. A heated humidifier can cost $500; the disposable, in-the-mask humidifiers cost about $5 each and reportedly work for up to two weeks.

Your health insurance may cover most, if not all, of the costs of CPAP. Talk to your insurance company to find out which equipment and supplies they will cover. (See Chap. 13 for more on selecting a CPAP.)

How Can You Obtain a CPAP?

You must have a doctor's prescription to obtain a CPAP. Your sleep center can put you in touch with a homecare company that will supply you with a CPAP system. The homecare company will send a respiratory therapist to your home to deliver the system and teach you how to operate it. They will provide same-day service in case of breakdown. (See Chaps. 13 and 14 on home-care companies.)

A few sleep centers rent or sell CPAP systems directly. However, most do not have the desire or the staff to deal with the paperwork and home service that this involves.

Other Air Pressure Devices

A couple of variations on the original CPAP mask are now available that replace the mask with a pair of small "pillows" or pads that rest against the nostrils. This device is less cumbersome than a face mask, and some people find it a more comfortable alternative.

Another refinement of CPAP is a two-level device called BiPAP™ by one manufacturer. This system allows the air pressure to be set and regulated at two different levels: the pressure delivered as the person exhales can be set to eliminate snoring, and the pressure delivered during exhaling can be set lower, making it easier to exhale.

Another variation on CPAP is a variable pressure system (called V-PAP by one manufacturer) that automatically adjusts pressure to accommodate to changes in breathing patterns that occur throughout the night.

These dual- and variable-pressure systems are becoming the treatment of choice for certain selected patients. At this writing the cost of such systems is two or more times that of CPAP, and for most people with sleep apnea the advantages probably would not justify (nor would insurance cover) the extra cost.

As you can see, the technology in this field is changing rapidly. If you are a candidate for CPAP, talk with the staff at your sleep center and with a homecare representative about the various versions of breathing devices that are available. You may want to test more than one and decide which one suits you best. (See Chap. 13 for more on choosing a CPAP.)

Oral Devices

A number of oral devices have been tried for treating sleep apnea. The objective behind the use of an oral device for sleep apnea is to hold the lower jaw, the tongue, or both in a forward position during sleep. Theoretically, this should keep the sleeper's airway open and prevent its collapse when the soft palate and tongue lose their muscle tone. Clearly, then, these devices are most likely to be effective for people whose obstructive apnea is caused primarily in the lower pharynx (throat), by the position of their tongue or lower jaw in relation to their airway.

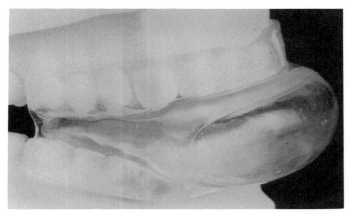

FIG. 7.4. A Samelson-type tongue-retaining device. The tongue is drawn forward into the bubble and held by suction.

The Tongue-Retaining Device

The *tongue-retaining device* (TRD) is made of soft plastic and consists of a tongue-sized suction cup that is supposed to pull the tongue forward and hold it in that position. It is gripped by the teeth and held in place during sleep (see Fig. 7.4).

Many of the people who have used the TRD in experiments have found it moderately uncomfortable to wear. For this reason in some experiments it was worn only half the night. Despite its drawbacks, the TRD was found to decrease the number of apnea events by approximately 50%. This means that the TRD could be about as effective as UPPP, a type of surgery described later.[23]

However, the TRD has not excited a lot of enthusiasm in the sleep research community and so far has not become widely used or available. Part of the reason for this is probably that the TRD apparently is useful only to a small group of obstructive apnea patients.

The people who are most likely to be helped by a TRD are those who are not obese, have no nasal obstructions, and have only slight to moderate apnea that is strongly influenced by sleeping position—that is, the apnea is much worse when sleeping on the back than when sleeping on the side.[24] For this group of people apnea apparently is strongly affected by tongue position;

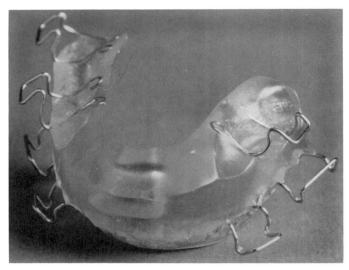

FIG. 7.5. A typical example of a jaw-retaining device. The metal loops hold the lower jaw in a forward position.

therefore holding the tongue forward with the TRD is supposed to be helpful. In some cases more severe apnea has been controlled with the use of a TRD.

Jaw Retainers

Another type of oral device that is being tested by several laboratories and sleep clinics is a jaw retainer. Actually, various retainer designs exist, all intended to hold the lower jaw forward.[25,26]

A jaw retainer looks like the bite plates or retainers that are sometimes prescribed by orthodontists. It is made of dental acrylic and usually has loops over several teeth that hold it in place. It must be custom-fitted. Some models contain small air tubes designed to equalize the air pressure inside and outside the mouth, thereby also, in theory, helping to prevent airway obstruction by preventing negative air pressure buildup in the back of the mouth (see Fig. 7.5).

Jaw retainers for sleep apnea are still experimental at the time of this writing. They may become more common if clinical trials can show that they are effective in eliminating apnea.

Who Can Benefit from Using a Jaw Retainer?

The manufacturers of jaw retainers and some experimenters who have patients using them have reported some good results[26]; however, jaw retainers do not help everyone.

Because jaw-retaining devices concentrate their treatment on the lower jaw and/or tongue, the people likely to have the best results are those with a smallish lower jaw that is set somewhat far back (called by orthodontists a Class II occlusion), plus moderate apnea. Retainers have been used successfully in children born with irregularly formed jaws who have difficulty with obstructive apnea.

People whose obstructive apnea comes mostly from nasal problems or from the upper pharynx (large tonsils, adenoids, soft palate, uvula) are less likely to be treated successfully with an oral device. In fact, you must be able to breathe through your nose to use the retainer; a person with a nasal obstruction or a stuffy nose from an allergy or a cold will be unable to wear one.

Some people who seem likely candidates for a jaw retainer continue to have apnea events, as shown by heavy snoring.

There may be a place for occasional use of an oral device. For example, (1) when CPAP is unavailable (backpacking, primitive travel); (2) when screening patients for mandibular advancement surgery (to simulate the possible results of surgery).

Getting Used to a Jaw Retainer

It may take from several nights to several weeks to get completely used to wearing a jaw retainer. Excess saliva will probably be an early side effect. Any foreign object in the mouth, such as a retainer, causes the production of excess saliva at first, but this generally tapers off after a night or two. However, it may take as long as two or three weeks for jaw muscles and other muscles to become accustomed to wearing a retainer. So the retainer may need to be worn that long in order to carry out a fair trial of the device and decide whether it is effective.

One disadvantage of the jaw retainer is that you can't rent one to try it out. You will not know whether a jaw retainer works for you until you have paid to have one made. However, if it works, you will be delighted. A jaw-retaining device is less restrictive of movement, much smaller, cheaper, and more convenient to deal with than a breathing device. If it doesn't work, other options are available.

How Much Do Jaw Retainers Cost?

Jaw retainers are cheaper than CPAP units, but still surprisingly expensive. Some manufacturers charge as much as $600. That is approximately twice the cost of an ordinary orthodontic retainer and does not include the cost of having your orthodontist or dentist take jaw impressions or the cost of additional visits to check or adjust the fit of the appliance. This can add another couple of hundred dollars to the cost. Check with your insurance company in advance to see if it will cover part or all of these costs.

Should You Try a Jaw Retainer?

If you and your sleep specialist feel you are a likely candidate for success with a jaw retainer, here are some questions to answer:
1. Have you had a sleep study to measure the baseline of your sleep apnea before treatment?
2. Is your sleep apnea mild?
3. If your sleep apnea is moderate to severe, have you tried CPAP (a more effective treatment)?
4. Can your sleep specialist refer you to a dentist who is experienced in fitting oral appliances for sleep apnea?
5. Do you have TMJ or dental problems that might be aggravated by using a jaw retainer?

6. Has your sleep specialist scheduled you for a follow-up sleep study, wearing the oral appliance, to verify its effectiveness?
7. Have you added up and talked with your insurance company about the full costs of an oral device, including fabrication, fitting, office visits for adjustments, and a follow-up sleep test? Do you consider this a cost-effective treatment option?

These questions are based partly on standards suggested by the American Sleep Disorders Association for the use of oral appliances.[27] Not everyone agrees with all the standards, but they offer important points for patients to consider when deciding upon their treatment.

Soon after you become adapted to using the oral appliance, you should return to the sleep center for a follow-up sleep study to determine whether the appliance is effectively eliminating your apnea. The sleep study must assess whether the retainer works both when you are sleeping on your back and when you are sleeping on your side.

Drugs for Treating Obstructive Sleep Apnea

So far drugs have not generally been shown to be very effective in treating obstructive sleep apnea. However, several of the drugs that have been tried unsuccessfully as treatments for central apnea (described earlier) have met with at least mixed success in obstructive apnea.

The hormone *medroxyprogesterone* has been found to be somewhat effective in some people with the Pickwickian syndrome. (See Chap. 8.) It has been reported to improve the breathing drive, to decrease the number of apnea events, and to improve the patient's symptoms.[8,28,29] However, some researchers have reported no improvement in apneas, so the results with this drug are conflicting.[6,8,29]

Medroxyprogesterone has some undesirable side effects. It can cause fluid retention, nausea, and depression in some people. Because it is a sex hormone, it can cause extra hair growth and breast tenderness. It should not be used by people with blood-clotting disorders or liver disease, by pregnant women, or by people known or suspected to have breast or genital cancer.

Protriptyline is an antidepressant that is variably effective in mild cases of sleep apnea. It is only a treatment option if the person's life is not in immediate danger from the effects of sleep apnea.

Drawbacks of protriptyline are that it decreases the amount of REM sleep and has a high incidence of other side effects: dry mouth, constipation (mild to intolerable), difficulty starting urine flow, and impotence.[28,30] It can cause confusion, especially in elderly people. It may be contraindicated (an undesirable treatment choice) for people with arrhythmias, very high blood pressure, glaucoma, or prostate disease.[29]

Other drugs have been tried as treatment for obstructive sleep apnea but have not been found to be effective.

Surgery

Surgery is the least conservative treatment for obstructive sleep apnea. It would be wise to consider other alternatives before this one is selected.

Four general types of surgery are used to treat obstructive sleep apnea:

❖ Nasal surgery.

❖ UPPP (uvulopalatopharyngoplasty).

❖ Mandibular (jaw) reconstruction and other maxillofacial procedures.

❖ Tracheostomy.

A fifth type of surgery has been used to eliminate snoring, but is not recommended for treating sleep apnea; however, we will discuss it in this chapter:

❖ LAUP (Laser Assisted Uvulopalatoplasty.

Nasal Surgery

Nasal surgery may actually refer to several different ear-nose-throat (ENT) procedures. These can include repair of the nasal septum (the wall that separates your left and right nasal passages), removal of polyps, surgery on the nasal sinuses, or submucous resection (removing loose tissue under the lining of the nasal passages).

By itself nasal surgery is not usually an effective treatment for sleep apnea or for snoring. Occasionally, some people report a decrease in snoring after surgery on their nose, only to have the symptoms return over several months.

For some people nasal surgery may be necessary to allow them to use CPAP. It may also permit them to wear an oral appliance that would have been impossible prior to surgery. A person who has poor airflow through his nose would feel suffocated wearing an oral appliance in his mouth.

Improved airflow through the nose can have a significant effect on overall airflow, and it should be considered as part of an overall surgical approach if UPPP (see the next section) is going to be carried out.

UPPP: Uvulopalatopharyngoplasty

UPPP is the most common type of reconstructive surgery done today for sleep apnea. It is basically plastic surgery on the soft palate and the inside of the throat. The throat wall is smoothed and tightened and excess tissue is removed (including tonsils, adenoids, and the uvula—the little tab that hangs down from the back of the roof of the mouth). The back of the soft palate is left in a streamlined shape that will be less likely to collapse during sleep.

Who Can Be Helped by UPPP?

Whether a person can be helped by UPPP depends on the reason for surgery and on how one defines being "helped." If the surgery is for purely "cosmetic" purposes (that is, simply to cut down on snoring), it stands about a 90% chance of being successful. Obviously, this type of improvement is measured by the bedpartner of the patient, and the opinion can be very subjective.

However, if the purpose of the surgery is to eliminate sleep apnea, then the chances of successful surgery are much more difficult to predict. In this case, the decision to have surgery is best reached after extensive discussion of the operation and the expected results with your sleep specialist and the ear-nose-throat (ENT) surgeon.

It is important to distinguish between an attempt to "help" sleep apnea and an attempt to "cure" sleep apnea (that is, eliminate all disease). UPPP surgery might "help" sleep apnea to varying degrees in different people. For example, Patients A and B might both show significant improvement after surgery. However, Patient A might need no further treatment, despite some remaining sleep apnea. (An example would be a person who goes from a sleepy patient with an RDI of 40 before surgery to an alert patient with an RDI of 10 after UPPP.) Patient B, on the other hand, might need further treatment after UPPP. (An example would be a person whose RDI of 60 improves to 30 after surgery but who still has low blood oxygen at night and is still drowsy.)

How often is sleep apnea "cured" by UPPP? That is difficult to say, but probably less than 20% of the time. Results like those of Patient A, who needs no further treatment, probably account for 20% to 40% of UPPP cases. Patients like Patient B, who needs treatment after surgery, probably account for 50% to 70% of UPPP cases.

People who are the most likely candidates for success with this type of surgery meet the following criteria:

1. They are not more than 25% or 30% over their ideal weight and they do not gain weight after surgery.[31,32]

2. They have only slight to moderate apnea, and it is all obstructive apnea.

3. Their apnea arises mostly from some obvious anatomic obstruction of the upper part of the pharynx (throat): the soft palate or upper throat area.[33,34] This includes people with enlarged tonsils or adenoids (tonsils and adenoids are customarily removed during UPPP), people with a very long soft palate or a large, fleshy uvula, and people with excess fleshy tissue in the throat region.

In contrast, people with very severe apnea or whose apnea arises from places other than the area of the soft palate are not good candidates for UPPP. Those with a lower jaw that is very

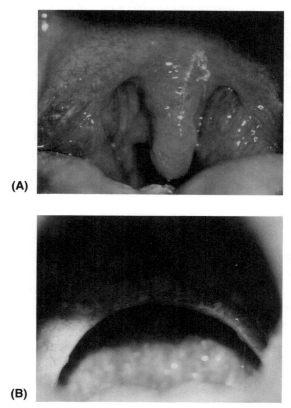

(A)

(B)

FIG. 7.6. UPPP surgery: **(A)** Before. Notice the large tonsils and fleshy uvula. **(B)** After. Tonsils and uvula have been removed.

short or placed far back, or with a tongue that is positioned fairly far back and low in the neck, or with apnea arising in the lower pharynx are less likely to be successful with UPPP.[34,35]

Body weight is an extremely important factor in the success of UPPP. The extra loading of the abdomen, which interferes with the breathing reflex, and the fatty deposits found in the neck, which help obstruct the airway, can both overpower any positive results that may be gained from UPPP. Therefore people who have UPPP and then gain weight are likely to see the return of their obstructive apnea.[31]

Until recently, not much was known about which people could best be helped by UPPP. With the aid of cephalometry (measurement of size and placement of structures in the head using x-ray, CAT scan, or MRI pictures) and fiberoptic examination of the inside of the airway, doctors are gradually gaining more information about how to choose the most likely candidates for successful UPPP.[35–39] Nevertheless, no one can predict the success of UPPP accurately.

Determining whether you are a good candidate for UPPP must be done by consulting with your sleep expert and a good otolaryngologist (ear-nose-throat specialist) who has experience not just with eliminating snoring but with sleep apnea problems. The otolaryngologist should examine your throat internally. He will probably order an x-ray, MRI, or CAT scan of your head so that he can measure the sizes and relationships between various anatomic features that cause your obstructive apnea. This will help him determine your chances of being helped by UPPP.

What Are the Drawbacks to UPPP?

UPPP is not a particularly risky kind of surgery, compared with many surgical procedures. It does not involve any large arteries or nerves. It may be performed as outpatient surgery in healthy, uncomplicated cases. In some patients one or two days in the hospital may be necessary.

The greatest risk, as mentioned earlier, is probably from the anesthesia. The more narrow the airway, the greater the risk from preoperative medications, from anesthetics, and from painkillers and sedatives given immediately after the operation.[1]

The reason for this increased risk is that anesthetics and some other drugs interfere with the breathing reflexes. If you have sleep apnea, you already have breathing reflexes that may not operate quite normally. This means that you are at somewhat greater than normal risk from anesthesia. This breathing abnormality, coupled with existing apnea, possible throat obstruction from postoperative swelling, and perhaps pain medication, could add up to serious complications in a person with breathing problems.

Pain is another consideration with UPPP. People who have had UPPP report that the pain after the operation is very severe— more painful than expected (for example, more painful than a tonsillectomy). Severe pain can last as long as a week.

All patients report difficulty swallowing after surgery. The removal of the uvula at the back of the mouth cavity makes it easier for material from the mouth to be pushed up into the back of the nasal cavity during swallowing. This is a common problem for the first two weeks after surgery, but it should correct itself with time, particularly if the surgeon is skilled and experienced with the procedure. A few people continue to have swallowing problems. However, most who do have a little difficulty swallowing find that with some practice, and if they eat properly, they overcome the problem.[1,32]

Why Have UPPP If the Odds Are Poor?

Even if the chances of being helped enough not to require further treatment are less than 50% to 60%, you may prefer taking a chance in the hope of avoiding other treatments, such as CPAP, oral appliances, or other surgeries.

When UPPP is performed on patients diagnosed at a top sleep center and the surgery is performed by one of their experienced ENT surgeons, the surgery has very low risk. (For example, at Providence Medical Center in Seattle there never has been a fatality or serious complication.)

How Can You Arrange for UPPP?

It is not advisable to have UPPP as a treatment for sleep apnea until you have been thoroughly examined by a physician who understands the causes of sleep apnea and knows how to weigh the benefits against the risks in your particular case. The sleep specialist, in turn, can refer you to a surgeon who is experienced with UPPP, if it appears that you are a good candidate for successful treatment by this procedure.

Maxillofacial Surgery

Maxillofacial surgery includes surgery on the mandible (lower jaw) and often the bones and tissue of the face and airway. These are not new surgeries, but they have a fairly short history of use as a treatment for sleep apnea, so in a sense they should be considered somewhat experimental.

The mandibular reconstruction surgery for treating sleep apnea actually includes some five or six possible surgical procedures. Various combinations of these procedures are done on different patients, depending on the different types of airway obstructions that they have. The surgeries include:

✤ Inferior sliding osteotomy (moves the lower jaw forward).

✤ Mandibular advancement (also moves the lower jaw forward).

✤ Hyoid myotomy.

✤ Hyoid resuspension (these latter two reposition the base of the tongue).

✤ Midface advancement (moves the upper jaw forward).

Several of these types of surgery have been practiced for some time by maxillofacial surgeons, who specialize in surgery

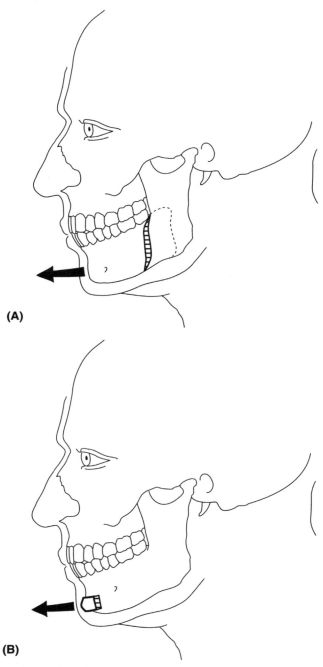

FIG. 7.7. Examples of mandibular and maxillofacial surgeries that have been tried for treating obstructive sleep apnea: **(A)** and **(B)**, two ways of pulling the lower jaw and the base of the tongue forward.

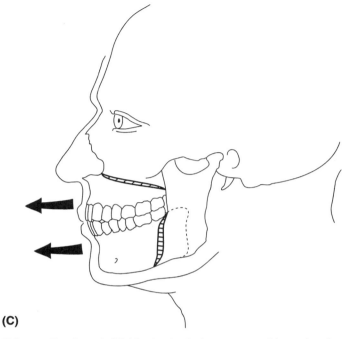

(C)

FIG. 7.7. Continued. **(C)** Moving both the upper and lower jaw forward.

involving the internal structures of the jaws and face. For example, lower jaw surgery is commonly done on people who have an unusually small or large lower jaw to bring the jaw into better proportion with the rest of the face and correct the bite. However, surgical procedures that reposition the base of the tongue are fairly new and still experimental (see Fig. 7.7).

Who Can Be Helped by Mandibular Advancement?

It is too early to be able to predict precisely who will be helped by maxillofacial surgery. More experience is needed with this type of surgery as a treatment for sleep apnea before such predictions can be made with assurance.

Mandibular advancement is the safest of these procedures and is being used more often nationally, although its usefulness is not yet fully established. It has been used only in a relatively small number of complicated apnea cases. An example is one patient who had a very small jaw and a small airway opening and for whom neither UPPP nor medication had helped. In this case, surgery did not completely eliminate his apnea, but it cut it about in half.[40] As with many examples of sleep apnea surgery, whether the results are successful or not depends on whether you define "success" as complete elimination of the apnea or whether you are satisfied with elimination of half of the apnea.

Among 1,000 people with obstructive apnea studied at one sleep center, about 6% had obviously malformed lower jaws, and another 32% had slightly short lower jaws.[41] It is among these people that the best candidates for mandibular advancement surgery would probably be found, because their apnea is likely to arise in part from structural problems in the lower pharynx: a jaw and tongue positioned further back and lower than normal, and an unusually small lower airway opening.

Mandibular surgery for sleep apnea should be planned as a team effort, involving the sleep specialist, an ear/nose/throat specialist, the maxillofacial surgeon who will perform the actual mandibular surgery, and an orthodontist if teeth are to be repositioned.[41]

The surgery itself is fairly safe if it is done by an experienced surgeon; however, it is performed under general anesthesia, which, as noted earlier, is especially risky for people with breathing disorders.

What Are the Drawbacks to Maxillofacial Surgery?

The main problem that can arise is difficulty with the healing of the jawbone, because the blood supply to that area is not very generous. The surgery presents a significant inconvenience to the patient, because it requires that the jaw be wired closed during healing for about six weeks. In addition, orthodontics may also be required to reposition the teeth and realign the bite. The entire procedure is expensive and time-consuming.

One further important drawback with this surgery should be considered. After mandibular surgery, the jawbone has a tendency to reposition itself backward again toward its original location. This happens over the course of several years, in response to the powerful force of the tongue muscles, which are constantly pulling on the jawbone. So although some surgeons would disagree, some other physicians have serious doubts about how long the results of this type of surgery will last.

Tracheostomy

Tracheostomy used to be a standard treatment for sleep apnea, but with the advent of CPAP, tracheostomy has become much less common. Today it is performed primarily on two types of patients: people who are very sick from the effects of sleep apnea and who need immediate (sometimes emergency) treatment to save their lives and those for whom other treatments have been unsuccessful. Tracheostomy has become the treatment of last resort; if all else fails, tracheostomy can be counted on to eliminate sleep apnea. In that sense it is a very hopeful form of surgery. It is also fairly simple.

What Is a Tracheostomy?

In a tracheostomy, a small opening is made into the trachea (windpipe), in the front of the neck just below the larynx (voice box). This opening may be considered permanent if tracheostomy is to be the permanent method of treating the person's sleep apnea. The opening can be surgically closed sometime in the future, if, for example, the patient switches to CPAP or some other treatment.

The idea of a tracheostomy is to allow air to bypass the obstructions in the upper airway. During waking hours the tracheostomy opening is closed with a plug and the person breathes normally through his nose and mouth. At night, however, the tracheostomy is left open and breathing is done through the neck opening, unobstructed.

A tracheostomy tube is usually worn in the tracheostomy opening. This is a small, curved tube with a flange at the top. It is inserted through the tracheostomy opening and extends a

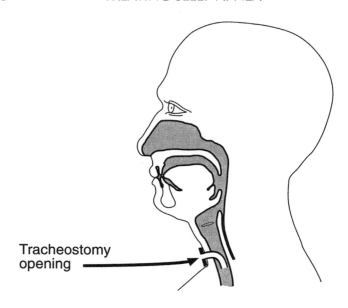

Tracheostomy
opening

FIG. 7.8. A tracheostomy, with tube in place. At night, the patient breathes through the tracheostomy opening, bypassing the obstruction in his airway. During the day, the tube is closed with a plug, so that the patient can talk.

couple of inches down into the windpipe. Usually, the tracheostomy tube is worn permanently. The flange at the top helps hold the tube in place and protects the opening in the throat (see Fig. 7.8).

Tracheostomy surgery itself is not particularly risky, although it is usually done under general anesthesia, and, as mentioned earlier, anesthesia can be risky. The complications that tend to arise with tracheostomy fall into two categories. One category involves the tracheostomy opening itself. In some cases the opening tries to close itself up again. Other difficulties can result if the tissue around the opening heals incorrectly or becomes infected, damaged, or eroded. To try to get around these kinds of problems, several different surgical variations have been developed. One variation is called a flap tracheostomy, in which the opening in the throat is lined with skin. This is supposed to eliminate the need for a tracheostomy tube.

Another set of complications of tracheostomy is respiratory infections such as pneumonia. When a person is breathing through a tracheostomy, he is breathing virtually straight into his lungs, bypassing all the natural germ-filtering systems in his nose and upper airway. Consequently, bacteria, viruses, and other foreign objects can much more easily reach the lungs. Great care must be taken to prevent this from happening.

After tracheostomy surgery there may be a fair amount of pain, some swelling, and difficulty swallowing for several days. Even after flap tracheostomy, a tracheostomy tube is worn until the incision has healed. The tube is chosen for size and shape to fit the particular person and is not particularly uncomfortable to wear.

After surgery, the patient and his family, and eventually the patient himself need to follow a fairly rigorous, 24-hour postoperative program of taking care of the tracheostomy. This includes cleaning, suctioning, misting, and applying salt solution and antibiotics. Immediately after surgery, a suction machine must be used periodically to keep the trach tube clear of mucous secretions that could block the airway. The suction machine will be needed indefinitely for cleaning the tube and preventing mucous buildup. As time goes on, mucous production decreases, so the frequency of suctioning also decreases. A humidifier can be used at night for the first several weeks after surgery to help keep mucous secretions from drying and blocking the tube. At all times, cleanliness will continue to be extremely important, to avoid introducing bacteria into the tracheostomy opening. The nurses and respiratory therapists should be explicit in teaching all these procedures to the patient and his family.

Who Can Be Helped by Tracheostomy?

Anyone with obstructive or mixed sleep apnea can be helped by a tracheostomy. Nowadays, the people chosen for tracheostomy, as mentioned earlier, usually have severe apnea with life-threatening complications, including excessive daytime drowsiness, to such a degree that they are completely disabled.[42]

They may have tried other treatments and found them unsuccessful. They may have significant arrhythmias or other serious heart complications from severe sleep apnea. They may have extremely low oxygen levels in their blood.

Tracheostomy eliminates snoring, improves the quality of sleep, and virtually cures daytime drowsiness and apnea in nearly everyone who has the surgery. It greatly improves fatigue and morning headaches.[42]

What Are the Drawbacks to Tracheostomy?

One of the main drawbacks of tracheostomy, and one reason it is falling out of favor so quickly with the advent of CPAP, is that depression is a common after-effect.

Most people need several weeks to months to learn to deal with the frustrations of tracheostomy hygiene and to adjust to their new image of themselves with a hole in their throat. A bout of depression commonly accompanies this adjustment period. The severity and duration of the person's depression (in fact, whether it occurs at all) depend on the individual, on how well the person has been prepared for the appearance and the care of the tracheostomy, and on the support of his family. The patient, his spouse, and other close family members should be counseled about the surgical procedure, the care that is necessary afterward, and the likelihood of some temporary depression. Talking with other people who have tracheostomies and are attending sleep apnea support groups, both before and after surgery, helps people to adjust more easily. (See the Appendix for some practical suggestions for living with a tracheostomy.)

Once the initial adjustment period is over, most people who have had tracheostomies report that they do just fine. They lead normal, active lives and generally do not seem to be bothered by their tracheostomies. However, they will always have to be careful about hygiene around the tracheostomy opening. And they must always take care that nothing gets into their windpipe through the tracheostomy opening. For example, people with tracheostomies cannot swim. Because the opening in their throat leads almost directly into the lungs, they are in extreme danger

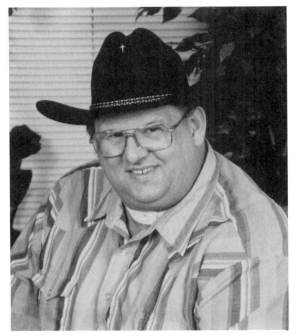

FIG. 7.9. This person has a tracheostomy.

from drowning. So people with tracheostomies must avoid not only swimming but all other water-related activities (water skiing, sailing, rafting, fishing from a boat) that might require swimming.

Other drawbacks involve the cosmetics of covering the tracheostomy opening. A small plate or shield is worn over the opening, held in place with a cord around the neck (see Fig. 7.9). There is nothing inherently objectionable about the appearance. However, many people choose to cover their tracheostomy plate with a turtleneck or a scarf. On some people the opening is up a little too high to be covered easily by clothing. One such patient recommended making a high-necked, elastic-topped dickey.[43]

Another problem can be keeping the opening sealed during the day. If there is air leakage, talking becomes difficult. Coughing or sneezing can sometimes pop the seal and cause temporary embarrassment.

Other difficulties, mentioned earlier, are problems that can arise from poor healing or erosion of the opening. To avoid such problems as these it pays to find the most skillful surgeon you can (consider a plastic surgeon) and to follow the postoperative instructions carefully. Ask your doctor to answer any questions you may have and be persistent in asking for help in learning to deal with any follow-up problems. (See the Appendix.)

Weight Loss Surgery (Gastric Bypass)

Weight loss surgery has been called "behavioral surgery,"[44] because it surgically enforces a change in the person's eating behavior that the person has been unable to accomplish by other means. The desired change in behavior is to reduce the amount of food the person consumes at any one sitting. Surgically, this is done by making the stomach smaller.

Several versions of weight loss surgery have been tried over the past 20 years. The most common procedure performed today is *gastric bypass.* In this surgery the stomach is reduced in size, not by removing part of the stomach, but by placing a row of staples across it, dividing the stomach into a small upper pouch and a larger lower pouch. The upper pouch becomes the "new" stomach. It receives food from the esophagus and empties into a branch of the intestines that has been brought up and attached to it.

After surgery, food intake at any one time will always be restricted to approximately twice the volume of the "new" stomach, which usually is about 30 ml. This means that no more than about one-quarter of a cup of food can be eaten at a time.

Gastric bypass is major surgery. It involves major organs (stomach and intestines), some large arteries, and the opening and closing of the abdominal cavity. There are risks from anesthesia and other medications. During and after surgery the placement of a number of tubes will add further to the invasiveness of the procedure: a nasogastric tube, for removing fluid from the stomach; catheters; intravenous hookups; possibly an endotracheal tube, for a ventilator. Gastric bypass surgery requires a hospital stay of a week or more, considerable postoperative pain and discomfort, and an extended recovery period lasting from four to five weeks to months.

Additional risk factors arise because this surgery is performed on people who are obese. For obese people the possibility of death from surgery is two to three times greater than that for people of average weight.[44] Consequently, it is important to weigh the risks carefully against the possible benefits that can reasonably be anticipated after surgery.

Complications after bypass surgery can be significant. They may include infections, bowel obstruction, collapse of lungs, blood clots, and other after-effects seen following abdominal surgery. (Obese people also have about twice the rate of postoperative complications, compared with people of ideal weight.)

The most common complication after gastric bypass is excessive vomiting.[44]

Who Can Be Helped by Gastric Bypass?

People who undergo this type of surgery are usually characterized as being "morbidly obese." The average weight of 17 patients in one group was *twice* their recommended body weight.[45] These are not people having cosmetic surgery to lose weight; these are people whose lives are in danger because of their excessive weight and other complications.

The patients chosen for gastric bypass are usually screened to include only those who have already made attempts to lose weight under carefully supervised weight loss programs. Often the patient's psychological status is evaluated as part of the screening process. Patients should understand the risks and the behavioral changes that will be necessary for the bypass surgery to be successful.

How Effective Is Gastric Bypass in Treating Apnea?

One study reported that, six months after surgery, most of their patients' sleep apnea was significantly improved. Some had completely lost their sleep apnea symptoms. Many patients reported no daytime sleepiness or loud snoring. Changes in personality were also reported: greater responsiveness, fewer emotional problems, less difficulty at work. A full year is needed for complete results, so during the six months following that report the patients in the study group might anticipate additional weight loss and further improvement in their apnea symptoms.[45] However, in the long term, some people who have had this surgery will return to their presurgery weight. The overall failure rate for gastric bypass surgery is reported to be 30% to 50%.[44]

In summary, for severely obese apnea patients who are motivated to change their eating behavior, gastric bypass surgery may be an effective and permanent, if radical, solution. The possible benefits should be weighed carefully against the significant potential risks.

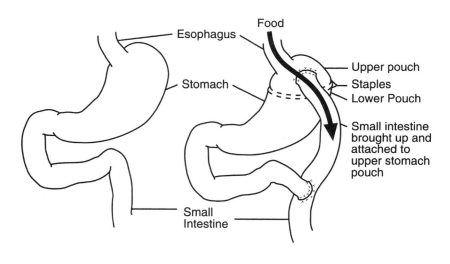

Normal   **Gastric Bypass**

FIG. 7.10. Gastric bypass surgery: the stomach is stapled crossways, which greatly reduces the amount of food it can hold. A loop of small intestine is attached to the upper stomach pouch to receive its contents.

Laser Surgery (LAUP) to Treat Snoring

Laser Assisted Uvulopalatoplasty (LAUP) is a technique for surgery on the soft palate that has been promoted recently as a harmless way to eliminate simple snoring. However, snoring is a symptom of sleep apnea, and LAUP has NOT been proven effective in treating sleep apnea.[46, 47]

The distinction between simple snoring and sleep apnea is not always clear. Frequently people who appear to have "simple snoring" turn out to have significant sleep apnea.[46] LAUP surgeons often try to screen out those patients with a questionnaire on snoring. However, such questionnaires tend to underestimate sleep apnea. Consequently many patients with undiagnosed sleep apnea have had LAUP surgery and have been left with a serious underlying disorder. To avoid unnecessary, possibly harmful LAUP surgery, people who snore should first be evaluated by a sleep specialist to rule out sleep apnea. Only after sleep apnea has been ruled out should people consider LAUP.

LAUP has also been promoted as a substitute for conventional palate surgery (UPPP, see pp. 106-111). Patients whose sleep and ENT specialist consider them good candidates for UPPP for treatment of snoring may want to consider LAUP for this purpose, but not to treat sleep apnea.

What Is LAUP?

LAUP involves several lengthwise laser "cuts" in a V-shaped pattern on the soft palate. Several sessions usually are needed. The laser cauterizes ("cooks") the tissue, leaving narrow scars which stiffen the tissue and presumably diminish the vibration that causes snoring.

Does LAUP Eliminate Snoring?

Proponents claim that it does in 80% to 90% of cases. Data still are insufficient to verify this success rate.

How Does LAUP Compare with Conventional UPPP?

LAUP is less risky: it involves less time, less bleeding, less tissue removal, no general anesthetic, and no hospitalization. It is somewhat cheaper (expect approximately $1,600 for surgeon, plus an additional fee for the surgical facility). Conventional UPPP involves a general anesthetic, a hospital stay, significant pain, plus risks from bleeding, infection, and general anesthetic. UPPP can cost approximately $3,000. However, the cost of UPPP is usually covered by insurance, while LAUP is not, at this writing.   Please read the sections in this chapter on choosing surgery in general, and on UPPP.

Can LAUP Treat Sleep Apnea?

No, it cannot, according to analyses published to date.[46]

The main danger from LAUP is that people who have a potentially fatal disorder, sleep apnea, may have LAUP under the mistaken impression that the surgery will cure them. Sleep apnea is more than snoring. (See Chap. 4, What Causes Sleep Apnea?)

The American Sleep Disorders Associations's standards of practice for LAUP recommend that patients be evaluated by a sleep specialist before LAUP. After surgery, people with sleep apnea should have a follow-up sleep study to determine whether the sleep apnea has been eliminated.[47]

Mr. Kennedy, the patient we have been following, finally reached the decision point: what treatment would be best for him?

When he first heard about UPPP, he thought it had some appeal: a relatively simple operation that might eliminate his snoring, and maybe his sleep apnea, for good. However, Mr. Kennedy's sleep specialist explained that he did not appear to be a very good candidate for UPPP. Mr. Kennedy has a short jaw, so most of his obstructive sleep apnea probably arises from low in his throat. It probably would not be resolved by UPPP. In that light, the pain and risks of surgery didn't seem worthwhile.

With the advice of his sleep specialist, Mr. Kennedy decided on CPAP combined with weight loss.

At the time this book is being written, Mr. Kennedy has been on CPAP for seven years. He lost 20 pounds and is at his ideal weight. He exercises several times a week, and feels better than he has ever felt in his life.

Mr. Kennedy travels a lot and takes his CPAP with him in a carry-on bag. Security people in airports often ask to look in the bag, but he has never been seriously hassled about it. Recently, he ran into an airport security guard who uses CPAP himself.

He has had occasional minor problems: colds, skin irritations, poorly fitting masks, equipment breakdown. But, like the pioneers that they are, Mr. Kennedy and other CPAP users learn to solve each problem as it arises.

Mr. Kennedy feels so much better now that he has never been seriously tempted to give up CPAP. He admits that he would rather not believe that he will have to use CPAP for the rest of his life. He was only 47 years old when he was diagnosed with sleep apnea, and he still thinks of himself as fairly young and vigorous. Sometimes he feels sorry to be saddled with this weird medical machine. But ... CPAP does work.

Maxillofacial surgery is Mr. Kennedy's only other option. So far he is not willing to trade the simplicity and effectiveness of CPAP for the risks, discomforts, and unpredictable results of surgery. Maybe some better treatment for sleep apnea will come along, someday. Meanwhile, he will stick with CPAP.

Summary

❖ *The best treatment is the most conservative treatment that will succeed for you.*

❖ *Treatments for central apnea:*

Medication.

Breathing devices such as mechanical ventilators and diaphragmatic pacemakers.

❖ *Treatments for obstructive sleep apnea and mixed apnea:*

Weight loss.

Breathing devices such as CPAP.

Oral devices such as tongue or jaw retainers.

Medication.

Surgery.

❖ *Before agreeing to surgery:*

Ask a qualified sleep specialist to estimate the chances that surgery will eliminate your sleep apnea.

Get a second opinion from an ENT surgeon who is experienced and skilled in the surgical treatment of sleep apnea.

➤ ➤ ➤ ➤ ➤ 8 ➤ ➤ ➤ ➤ ➤ ➤

Obesity and Sleep Apnea ·

SIMPLE OBESITY AND OBSTRUCTIVE SLEEP APNEA

Obesity is defined as being 20% heavier than your ideal weight as a result of excess body fat.

Not everyone with sleep apnea is obese, nor does everyone who is obese have sleep apnea. However, there is a strong correlation between the two.

THE SINKING SPIRAL

The reasons obesity and sleep apnea tend to go hand in hand are threefold:

1. In obesity fatty deposits accumulate within the layers of tissue in the neck. This causes constriction of the airway.
2. In obese people excess fatty tissue in the abdomen causes abnormal loading that interferes with the normal breathing reflex.
3. A sinking spiral develops, involving reduced activity and increased weight. As sleep apnea worsens, EDS (excessive daytime sleepiness) also worsens. The person becomes less active, uses less energy, gains more weight, and further aggravates the apnea.

The key to treatment is to break the cycle. For some people, weight loss alone can effectively do this. However, weight loss may be difficult or impossible to achieve as long as the sleep apnea is untreated.

Case Study. Mrs. Baker had gained 50 pounds and felt increasingly exhausted. Her sleep was restless and unrefreshing, and her terrible, irregular snoring concerned her husband because she appeared to be gasping for breath. Her doctor told her to lose weight and refused to refer her to a sleep center because "that's what they will tell you to do anyway."

Mrs. Baker joined a weight loss program and lost 50 pounds, after spending $3,000. Her snoring improved a great deal but did not go away; and although her exhaustion had largely disappeared, she still felt drowsy when sitting, reading, or relaxing. Within seven months her excess weight had returned, and with it her symptoms.

Another physician agreed to refer her to a sleep center. Moderately severe sleep apnea was diagnosed. Mrs. Baker was placed on CPAP, which eliminated her sleep apnea. On CPAP and with the help of a dietitian she again lost the weight. Now at her ideal weight, she was again studied at the sleep center. To her dismay, unless she slept with CPAP, she still had 50% of her sleep apnea.

Looking back, Mrs. Baker realized that after her initial and expensive weight loss, her apnea had continued to leave her fatigued and had decreased her activity level. As a result, her weight had increased; and as she saw herself failing, she became depressed and ate more.

Now, using CPAP, Mrs. Baker is able to maintain her new weight.

CPAP eliminates the obstructive apnea, allowing more restful sleep and better blood oxygen, which boost the person's energy level. The increase in energy and activity can then contribute to the weight loss effort.

THE PICKWICKIAN SYNDROME

The Pickwickian syndrome is a special type of sleep apnea that is associated with overweight. It is essentially severe sleep apnea combined with obesity and a chronically decreased breathing pattern called *hypoventilation*. This syndrome is found in about 5% of sleep apnea patients.[1]

Case Study. Mr. Roberts is a 45-year-old computer programmer and former college track star. He had always been an active, energetic man with lots of outside interests.

It was 1979 when Mr. Roberts first became aware that something was wrong with him. He realized that he felt tired a lot of the time. He had no energy. He became less and less active, and he started to gain weight. He began to take a lot of naps. Eventually, he was falling asleep at work. Fortunately, his boss liked and respected him and was sympathetic, although puzzled. He wondered if Mr. Roberts had a problem with alcohol or drugs and hoped that in time he would be able to work it out.

Between 1979 and 1985, Mr. Roberts changed from a trim, fun-loving, lively man into an overweight, lethargic, crabby near-invalid. He was asleep, or half asleep, nearly all the time. He had also developed heart problems. His doctor was stumped.

Mrs. Roberts was desperately worried. One day she heard by chance about a new sleep disorder center and talked her reluctant husband into making an appointment.

The sleep specialist recognized Mr. Roberts's problem immediately as a variety of sleep apnea. From the information in Chapter 1 you may recognize in Mr. Roberts one of the most common symptoms of sleep apnea: excessive daytime sleepiness.

Some clues from Mr. Roberts's past might have tipped you off further: his ability to fall asleep anywhere in any position and his loud snoring. When he was in the service, he was legendary: his snoring was so horrendous that his buddies often had to carry him outside in the middle of the *night so that they could get some sleep. Many a morning Mr. Roberts woke up on his cot in the middle of the parade ground.*

By the time he visited a sleep clinic, Mr. Roberts was showing all the symptoms of the Pickwickian syndrome.

For centuries observers have linked obesity, breathing disorders, and drowsiness. Dionysius, the Tyrant of Heracleia during the time of Alexander the Great, was described by historians as extremely obese and continually sleepy and was said to have had difficulty breathing. In fact, he is reported to have been "choked by his own fat." Magas, king of Cyrene, also obese, was also said to have "choked himself to death" in 258 B.C.

In 1816 William Wadd, surgeon to King George III of England, connected obesity, lethargy, and breathing difficulty. He described three patients who were "suffocated by fat." And in 1889 another medical man, A. Morison, reported a case of an obese, drowsy man whose drowsiness improved after he lost weight.[2,3]

It was not until the 1950s that anyone came close to explaining what causes the Pickwickian syndrome. A respiratory physiologist was the first to suggest a cause-and-effect link between obesity and breathing difficulty. He proposed that obesity places an extra load on the respiratory system and suggested that this leads to lethargy and sleepiness.[2] But he failed to connect sleep apnea with the total picture. Finally, in 1965 Gastaut demonstrated the relationship between sleep apnea and excessive daytime sleepiness.

The term *Pickwickian* was first used as a medical term in an article by Bramwell in 1910. One of his patient's symptoms reminded him of the description and behavior of the fat boy, Joe, in Dickens' *The Posthumous Papers of the Pickwick Club* (1837). In Dickens' words:

A most violent and startling knocking was heard at the door; it was...a constant and uninterrupted succession of the loudest single raps, as if the knocker were endowed with the perpetual motion, or the person outside had forgotten to leave off.

Mr. Lowton hurried to the door....The object that presented itself to the eyes of the astonished clerk was a boy—a wonderfully fat boy—...standing upright on the mat, with his eyes closed as if in sleep. He had never seen such a fat boy,...and this, coupled with the utter calmness and repose of his appearance, so very different from what was reasonably to have been expected of the inflicter of such knocks, smote him with wonder.

"What's the matter?" inquired the clerk.

The extraordinary boy replied not a word; but he nodded once, and seemed, to the clerk's imagination, to snore feebly.

"Where do you come from?" inquired the clerk.

The boy made no sign. He breathed heavily, but in all other respects was motionless.

The clerk repeated the question thrice, and receiving no answer, prepared to shut the door, when the boy suddenly opened his eyes, winked several times, sneezed once, and raised his hand as if to repeat the knocking. Finding the door open, he stared about him with astonishment, and at length fixed his eyes on Mr. Lowton's face.

"What the devil do you knock in that way for?" inquired the clerk, angrily.

"Which way?" said the boy, in a slow, sleepy voice.

"Why, like forty hackney-coachmen," replied the clerk.

"Because master said I wasn't to leave off knocking till they opened the door, for fear I should go to sleep," said the boy.

To anyone who has no experience with the Pickwickian syndrome, this scene may seem far-fetched. But Dickens was a keen observer of humankind, and clearly depicted the most obvious symptoms:

✤ Marked obesity.

✤ Daytime drowsiness.

✤ Tendency to fall asleep during routine activities.

✤ Snoring.

Other features of the Pickwickian syndrome that are less obvious to the casual observer are:

✤ Sleep apnea.

✤ Bluish tone to face (cyanosis).

✤ Abnormal breathing reflexes.

✤ Enlargement of right side of the heart.

✤ Heart failure.

What Causes the Pickwickian Syndrome?

The Pickwickian syndrome is the result of several conditions coming together at once: sleep apnea, an abnormal breathing pattern, obesity, and usually some obstructive lung disease.[1] However, it is not completely clear which condition first causes which.

Apparently, Pickwickian people have a built-in tendency for a slightly abnormal breathing reflex, which gradually can become less sensitive to the amount of the waste gas, carbon dioxide, in the blood. (See Chap. 3.) If this tendency is combined with sleep apnea, the result is low oxygen and high carbon dioxide levels in the blood at night (and, in some people, continuing into daytime as well), and disturbed sleep.

These factors, in turn, lead to daytime sleepiness, a characteristic result of sleep apnea. As obesity is added to the picture, additional problems arise, as described earlier: excess weight in the abdomen further perturbs the breathing reflexes[4,5]; and extra fatty tissue in the neck constricts the airway.

The Pickwickian syndrome can begin in childhood, or it can occur in adults who formerly were quite thin.

What Are the Effects of the Pickwickian Syndrome?

The Pickwickian syndrome leads to the same problems that result from other kinds of sleep apnea. A Pickwickian person has fragmented sleep. Deep sleep and REM sleep are reduced, sometimes nearly to zero. And because he does not take in sufficient oxygen during the night, he suffers from a kind of slow asphyxiation.[4,6]

Excessive drowsiness during the daytime is common. Pickwickian people have a remarkable tendency to fall asleep whenever there is a moment's relaxation. They often fall asleep at their desks at work, in the middle of a conversation, or while driving a car.

Mr. Roberts tells of habitually driving to work and falling asleep in the parking lot. His coworkers would come out and find him, turn off the car, and guide him in to his office, where he would spend the day sleeping at his desk. A Pickwickian doctor reported dozing off while examining a patient. He awoke to find his head resting on the patient's shoulder. A Pickwickian business executive finally sought treatment after falling asleep during a weekly poker game—he had drawn a full house (aces over kings) but then dropped off to sleep and missed the play.[7]

Serious heart disease is closely associated with the Pickwickian syndrome.[4,6,7] In addition to the risks of hypertension, stroke, and coronary artery disease that accompany obesity, there are the risks of heart enlargement, arrhythmias, pulmonary complications, and heart failure that can result from sleep apnea. There is a relatively high rate of sudden death among the obese.[6] The Pickwickian syndrome should be treated seriously, because in the long term it is certainly life-threatening.

Treating the Pickwickian Syndrome

CPAP combined with weight loss is the most conservative treatment. If CPAP is not able to eliminate the sleep apnea and low blood oxygen, a temporary tracheostomy may be used. (See Chap. 7.)

The medical reports are mixed in their opinions about the effectiveness of weight loss in reducing the symptoms of this syndrome. However, it may be that the more weight lost, the more likely it is that the person's apnea will improve. For any particular individual there may be a critical weight, above which the breathing difficulties of the Pickwickian syndrome appear. Below that weight improvement can be expected.[7]

The combination of CPAP (to eliminate the apnea, the oxygen deprivation, and the debilitating daytime drowsiness) and a serious long-term weight loss program can have dramatic results. Mr. Roberts is a good example.

Case Study (continued). Mr. Roberts was put on CPAP and a weight loss program. A year after beginning treatment for sleep apnea, Mr. Roberts was quite literally a different person. He had lost 100 pounds and was full of energy. He continued to lose weight steadily and was working at regaining his health. Thanks to a sympathetic boss, he still had his job. He was also remodeling his house (doing much of the work himself) and restoring several classic cars. He didn't have time to take naps.

Some Pickwickian people treated in this way appear to have a complete "remission." They can stop using CPAP, and they appear to be cured of sleep apnea.[8]

Weight loss surgery (gastric bypass) is reported to be effective in treating the Pickwickian syndrome, reducing sleep apnea to near zero and restoring deep sleep and REM sleep.[6] However, gastric bypass surgery is not a trivial operation, and this should not be considered a conservative treatment option. (See Chap. 7 for further information on treatment of sleep apnea.)

Summary

❖ *Obesity is common among obstructive apnea patients.*

❖ *The Pickwickian syndrome is a form of sleep apnea caused by a combination of obesity, obstructive apnea, and an abnormal breathing reflex.*

❖ *Symptoms of the Pickwickian syndrome include:*

　Obesity.

　Daytime drowsiness.

　Falling asleep during routine activities.

　Snoring and sleep apnea.

❖ *Treatments include CPAP and weight loss.*

➤➤➤➤➤ 9 ➤➤➤➤➤

Sudden Infant Death Syndrome and Sleep Apnea in Infants

IS SLEEP APNEA THE CAUSE OF SUDDEN INFANT DEATH SYNDROME?

Is sleep apnea the cause of sudden infant death syndrome (SIDS)? Probably not, but the answer depends a lot on how SIDS is defined. SIDS is considered a sleep disorder, but its exact cause (or causes) is still unknown and somewhat controversial.

Whenever a condition is identified as a cause of infant death, it immediately falls under scrutiny as potentially *the* cause of SIDS. Some researchers believe this is what happened a few years ago when sleep apnea was advanced as the possible cause of SIDS. However, other researchers believe there is mounting recent evidence to link SIDS to obstructive sleep apnea.[1]

One authority has compared the current understanding of SIDS to a table littered with jigsaw puzzle pieces. "Our task is to fit [the pieces] together and to identify how many pieces are missing. One difficulty is that we don't know how many different jigsaw puzzles the pieces belong to."[2]

The question remains: are sleep apnea and SIDS completely separate jigsaw puzzles whose pieces have gotten mixed together? Some of the pieces seem to fit, but do they really belong to the same puzzle? In other words, some infants die from SIDS and some infants die from apnea, but they may not be dying for the same reasons.

SLEEP APNEA IN INFANTS

Variations in breathing during sleep are common, and even normal, in infants. As explained by one authority: in infants "pauses in breathing are an integral part of normal respiratory behavior, are strongly influenced by age and sleep state, and do not of themselves constitute an abnormality."[3]

Premature infants tend to have more and longer apnea events than full-term infants. This is because premature infants still have immature breathing reflexes.[4] Normally, apnea in premature infants is not considered a problem unless the apnea events appear to be prolonged.

In a normal, full-term infant, apnea during sleep is common. It is most common shortly after birth and decreases with age. However, frequent or prolonged apnea events are not normal and may be a sign of a breathing problem that should be called to the attention of a doctor. Experts disagree as to how much apnea should be considered a danger sign. Two or more apnea events of more than 20 seconds during an eight-hour period would be considered prolonged apnea.[3] Infants showing this kind of apnea during their first month of life might be considered at higher risk from apnea and may need to be watched carefully.

APNEA OF INFANCY VERSUS "NEAR-MISS SIDS"

Infants who have been found not breathing, and blue, are often called "near-miss SIDS" infants: if they had not been resuscitated, their deaths would have been attributed to SIDS. However, since the actual cause of SIDS is unknown, the label *near-miss SIDS* is misleading. These infants' apnea may be entirely unrelated to whatever causes SIDS.

Sometimes the cause of these infants' breathing failure can be pinpointed. Many factors can cause apnea in infants: congenital heart or lung abnormalities, structural abnormalities of the face or upper airway, bacterial or viral infections, sedatives, seizures, and possibly reflux (regurgitation of stomach contents). The presence of any of these factors may increase the likelihood of a breathing problem during sleep.[5]

When an infant's apnea doesn't seem to be related to any of these causes, the diagnosis is simply *apnea of infancy*, which is a more accurate term than *near-miss SIDS*.

Infants with unexplained apnea of infancy probably should be given a polygraphic sleep test to try to determine the cause and severity of the apnea.

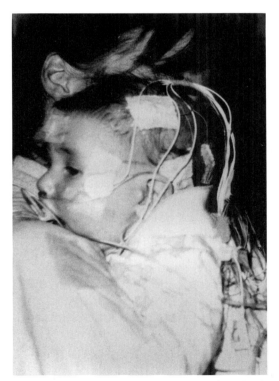

FIG. 9.1. A child who is suspected of having a sleep disorder is prepared for a sleep test at a sleep center.

RISK FACTORS FOR SIDS

Two groups of infants have been thought to be at risk for SIDS:

1. Near-miss SIDS infants (infants with apnea of infancy).
2. Subsequent siblings of SIDS victims.

Studies have shown that infants in these two groups have a greater likelihood of SIDS than other infants.

However, these two groups of infants account for only a very small portion of the total number of SIDS victims.[5] So, clearly, serious breathing problems may increase the risk for SIDS, but many other factors must be involved.

If you have an infant whom you feel may fall into a higher-risk category, you may want to talk to your pediatrician about your concern and ask for a consultation with a sleep specialist.

APNEA MONITORS: COPING WITH RISK

What can be done when an infant appears to be at risk for apnea? One possibility is to use an electronic apnea monitor. A number of apnea monitors are available that can be used at home. However, they are not totally effective.

An apnea monitor consists of a sensor that is either placed under the baby's mattress or attached to the baby's abdomen. If breathing stops for a selected period of time, usually 20 seconds, the monitor signals the parents by ringing a bell and flashing a light. The monitors are not foolproof, however. They can give false positive alarms, sometimes as often as 25% to 50% of the time. A lot of false alarms can be discouraging for the parents and may tempt them to turn off the monitor.[6]

More serious is the fact that monitors can also give a false negative response. That is, they can fail to indicate that breathing has stopped, when it has. This can happen if the baby stops breathing, but the heartbeat, which becomes stronger when breathing stops, is still felt by the monitor. Also, in obstructive apnea, when breathing stops but abdominal muscle movements are still being made against the obstruction, the monitor may misinterpret these as breathing. In either case the alarm might not go off until all motion has stopped, by which time brain damage or death may have occurred.[6]

Despite these drawbacks there are cases in which a monitor might be helpful: for a premature infant who seems susceptible to prolonged apnea events; for a "near-miss" infant who already has been found apneic (not breathing), blue, and limp (although this can have numerous causes, so the infant should be examined first); and for some siblings of SIDS victims who are considered to be high risk and whose parents need reassurance.[6]

The monitor should be used for as long as the physician and parents feel it is necessary. This may be from three to five months, until the child reaches an age the physician regards as safely beyond the risk of SIDS. Or the physician may wait until the child passes through an adequate alarm-free period and appears able to tolerate immunizations and respiratory infections without breathing difficulty.[5]

If an apnea monitor is going to be used, the baby should be examined by a physician familiar with these devices, in order to decide upon the best type of monitor to use. In addition, a 24-hour support service should be arranged, through the doctor or the hospital, in case of equipment breakdown. Finally, parents *must* be trained in methods of resuscitation. In fact, resuscitation training (CPR) should be given to any parents whose child is considered to be at risk for SIDS or apnea attacks. If you feel you need such training, ask your doctor to arrange it for you or ask your local Red Cross for a schedule of their classes.

TREATING INFANT SLEEP APNEA

Most infant apnea disappears as the infant matures. If this is not the case, various treatment options, including nasal CPAP, may be suggested by a sleep specialist, depending on the cause of the apnea (see Fig. 9.2).

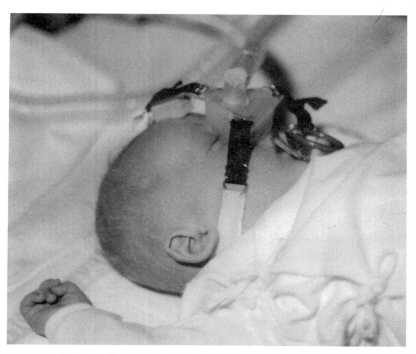

FIG. 9.2. A six-week-old infant being treated with CPAP, wearing a ResCare Bubble Mask™.

Summary

❖ Sleep apnea can result in infant death but may not be the cause of most cases of Sudden Infant Death Syndrome (SIDS).

❖ Infants diagnosed as having "apnea of infancy," or who are younger siblings of SIDS infants, are at higher risk from SIDS.

❖ Infants with "apnea of infancy" should receive a thorough evaluation, including a sleep study.

❖ For high-risk infants use of an apnea monitor may be indicated.

❖ Treatment depends on the cause of the sleep apnea, as discussed in the chapter.

❖ Consult a sleep specialist if you suspect sleep apnea in an infant.

➤➤➤➤➤ 10 ➤➤➤➤➤

Sleep Apnea in Older Children and Adolescents

Sleep apnea in older children is probably more common today than it was a generation ago. This is because tonsillectomies are much less common now, so many more children today have enlarged tonsils and adenoids. Enlarged tonsils or adenoids are the main causes of sleep apnea in children.[1]

> **Case Study**. *Jody was a ten-year-old who had been snoring terribly for three years. She also made snorting noises in her sleep. During the day, both at home and at school, she was tired and short-tempered. Her tonsils were large, but her pediatrician did not believe in taking out tonsils unless they were regularly becoming infected. He told the family she would outgrow this.*
>
> *The family physician suggested an evaluation at a sleep center. The sleep test revealed that Jody had severe apnea, with 40 apnea events per hour. She had a tonsillectomy, her symptoms disappeared, and her temper and her school grades improved markedly.*

CAUSES OF SLEEP APNEA IN CHILDREN

The causes of sleep apnea in children are similar to the causes of apnea in adults:

❖ Central apnea, the result of an abnormal breathing reflex.

❖ Obstructive apnea, the result of a narrow or blocked airway. Airway blockage can arise from nasal obstruction resulting from a deviated septum or from allergies, large tonsils or adenoids, large soft palate, small lower jaw, and other structural features of the mouth, jaw, or throat that result in a narrow upper airway. Obesity is also a contributing factor.

❖ Mixed apnea, a combination of central and obstructive apnea.

SYMPTOMS OF SLEEP APNEA IN CHILDREN

The symptoms of sleep apnea in children often are somewhat different from those seen in adults. Drowsy children may behave differently from drowsy adults. Children whose apnea arises primarily from obesity are most likely to have the signs you would expect in an adult.[1]

Snoring is the most obvious symptom: heavy snoring, accompanied by loud snorting, alternating with silence, is a sign of fairly severe obstructive apnea. A less complete obstruction might sound like lighter snoring alternating with heavy breathing.

Restless sleep and *unusual sleep positions* are other possible signs of sleep apnea. Often a child who is having trouble breathing will thrash about, sit up, or kneel and bend forward in a position that helps to keep his airway open.

Daytime sleepiness is one sign of sleep apnea that may appear differently in children and adults. An adult who suffers from excessive daytime sleepiness will normally seem fatigued or sleepy. A child may instead seem *irritable, aggressive* or *hyperactive*, or *forgetful*, or *"lazy."* Or the child may simply appear *quiet, withdrawn,* or pathologically *shy.* His "good" behavior may not be perceived as a sign of a problem, even by his family.

Poor performance at school—poor concentration, underachievement, behavioral problems—is one of the most typical signs of sleep apnea. It is estimated that two-thirds of the children who are eventually diagnosed as having sleep apnea are not recognized until their parents are alerted to a problem by school authorities.

Other possible signs of sleep apnea are *bedwetting, morning headaches,* and *cardiovascular problems,* such as high blood pressure and arrhythmias (heartbeat abnormalities).

Untreated sleep apnea in children is likely to become worse and in time leads to the same kinds of cardiovascular and respiratory complications as are seen in adults. In the long term it should be considered life-threatening. Furthermore, it is impossible to overstate the disadvantages these children may suffer as a result of poor performance in school. The consequences of poor concentration and behavioral problems can affect a child for the rest of his life, so no time should be lost in treating sleep apnea.

If your pediatrician or family physician is not familiar with sleep apnea, he may fail to recognize its signs. You might want to make a tape recording of the sounds of your child's snoring and ask your doctor to refer you to a sleep specialist. It is important that a child who is suspected of having sleep apnea be tested thoroughly by a sleep specialist and that treatment be scheduled as soon as possible.

TESTING FOR SLEEP APNEA IN CHILDREN

As with adults, diagnosis of sleep apnea and other sleep disorders (see Chap. 6) is most effectively done in an accredited sleep center. The following two cases have similar symptoms and show that inadequate testing can easily lead to misdiagnosis and inappropriate treatment.

Case Study. Becky was eight and had been waking up yelling and shaking her legs rhythmically. She was tired and appeared confused the next day. This happened a few times a month and was very disturbing to her parents. They took her to a neurologist, but nothing was found. She was then studied in a sleep center and was found to have a seizure disorder. Her parents agreed to start her on medications, and her episodes stopped entirely.

Case Study. *Mary was seven and had been waking up moaning, with her legs rigid and shaking. She appeared confused, and her parents thought she looked as if she were having seizures. Her neurologic evaluation was negative, but she had some "abnormalities" in her EEG. She was diagnosed as having seizures and was given medications. She developed a severe rash. Eventually, her parents took her to a sleep center, where she was diagnosed as having a night terror disorder that mimicked seizures. She was treated with counseling and her spells gradually disappeared.*

Diagnostic testing for sleep apnea in children should include a thorough physical exam, with special emphasis upon the anatomy of the face, neck, and upper airway. This may include a fiberoptic examination of the airway.

An x-ray-type image of the child's head may also be needed. This can by done using several techniques, each of which has drawbacks. X-ray exams (roentgenograms) and fluoroscopic examinations will expose the child's head to ionizing radiation, which poses a significantly greater hazard for children than for adults. Computerized tomography (CAT scan, especially fast CT) is less hazardous, and MRI (magnetic resonance imaging) is harmless, but both of these procedures are more expensive. Consult with your doctor about which of these options is most appropriate.

An overnight sleep test should be performed to confirm the presence of sleep apnea, to measure the severity of the disorder, and to rule out other disorders. A multiple sleep latency test (MSLT) should also be done to measure the degree of sleepiness.

The results of a child's sleep test may be evaluated a little differently from those of an adult. Very little is known about how much apnea occurs in normal children, so it is difficult to know how much apnea should be considered "abnormal." In adults an apnea index greater than five apneas per hour of sleep is considered a sign of sleep apnea. Some sleep experts believe that a respiratory disturbance index (RDI, apneas plus hypopneas) of 5 is high for a child.[2]

Because adults and children with sleep apnea differ in both symptoms and sleep test results, it would be wise to look for a sleep specialist who is experienced with pediatric sleep disorders.

TREATING OBSTRUCTIVE SLEEP APNEA IN CHILDREN

Since most obstructive apnea in children arises from enlarged tonsils and adenoids, the most frequent treatment is simply to remove them. The operation has some risk but is fairly routine.

In adults several other types of surgery have been used to treat sleep apnea. These surgeries usually are not appropriate in a child. Because the child's bones and soft tissues are still growing, there is a chance the obstructive apnea may disappear as growth occurs.

Medications are another treatment sometimes used in adults. The drugs used in adults either are generally inappropriate in children or have not been found to be very effective.

CPAP is becoming the treatment of choice for children whose obstructive sleep apnea is not or cannot be resolved by tonsillectomy. Children with abnormally small jaw structure may be placed on CPAP until they are old enough (teenage) for surgery to be effective. In young children CPAP is most successful when the child is able to understand how the mask and CPAP equipment work and when the parents are cooperative.[3] CPAP is well tolerated by teenagers.

If obesity is part of the problem, weight loss is usually helpful. Weight loss works best if the whole family is involved in a program of weight loss and counseling.[1] Extremely severe apnea may need corrective surgery, such as UPPP or mandibular surgery, as described in Chapter 7.

Regardless of treatment, a follow-up sleep study is a good idea to confirm that the therapy has been effective.

SUMMARY

❖ Sleep apnea in older children usually arises either from enlarged tonsils or adenoids or from obesity.

❖ Consult a sleep specialist if you suspect sleep apnea in a child. The diagnosis can be tricky because symptoms of sleep apnea in children may not appear to be related to sleep.

❖ Treatment depends on the cause of the sleep apnea, as discussed in the chapter.

>>>>> 11 >>>>>

Sleep Apnea and the Senior Citizen

SLEEP IN OLDER PEOPLE

We often assume that it is normal for older people to get less sleep during the night than younger people. This assumption is often explained by the further assumption that "older people don't need as much sleep." In fact, both of these assumptions are open to question.

It is true that people over 50 typically do get about six hours of sleep during the night, compared with eight hours for people 19 to 30 years old. This is partly because older people awaken more often during the night and partly because they usually wake up earlier in the morning.[1] However, older people also appear to take more frequent daytime naps than young people. So an older person's total *amount* of sleep during a 24-hour period may be very close to the eight hours obtained by a younger person.[2]

However, the *quality* of sleep that older people get is not as good as it is in younger people. From reading Chapter 3 you know that when a night's sleep is broken up by wakefulness, the quality of the sleep is diminished. Older people's sleep is lighter and more fragmented by periods of wakefulness than the sleep of younger people. In Fig. 11.1 you can see these differences by comparing the pattern of sleep in a young adult with that of an older person.

A

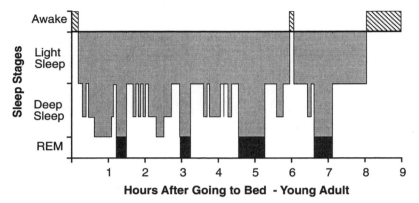

Hours After Going to Bed - Young Adult

B

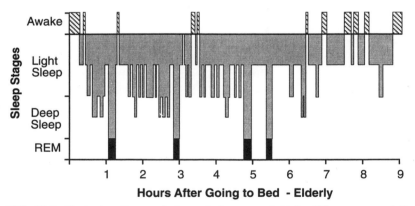

Hours After Going to Bed - Elderly

FIG. 11.1. Typical patterns of sleep during one night for **(A)** a young adult and for **(B)** an elderly person. The young adult has more deep sleep and longer REM periods. The older person has more shallow, broken sleep and shorter REM periods.

Older people get less deep sleep (see Fig. 11.2). They get almost as much REM sleep as younger people, but it is less intense.[1]

By napping, older people may be attempting to compensate for sleep lost during the night. In some individuals naps may make up for the amount of sleep lost. However, they do not make up for the loss of sleep quality at night. In fact, in some people naps may simply compound the problem, both by making the person less sleepy at night and by confusing the person's internal clock.

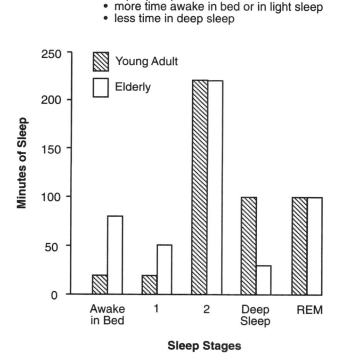

FIG. 11.2. Comparison of the amount of time young people and older people spend in each stage of sleep.

The significance of these differences between older and younger people's sleep is not understood. No one knows exactly why we need deep sleep and REM sleep, so the meaning of the decrease in these stages of sleep with age remains to be discovered.

MYTHS ABOUT SLEEP AND AGING

The majority of older people are healthy and have few, if any, complaints about sleep disturbances. Even though their sleep may be more fragmented than it was when they were younger, they do not appear to be unduly bothered by it. However, some older people do have serious sleep problems. Unfortunately, they may be discouraged from seeking help by certain myths about sleep and aging.

❖ Feeling sleepy is *not* "just part of getting old." Do not accept this explanation by family physicians, or even your own rationalizations that tell you that being sleepy during the day is "just part of being old." If you are drowsy to the point that it affects your ability to drive alertly for at least an hour, to read for 30 or more minutes, or to sit and socialize with family, the odds are that you may have a treatable sleep disorder.

❖ Disturbed or poor sleep is *not* normal. Do not accept explanations that say that disturbed or poor nighttime sleep is "normal." Although most elderly people would agree that their sleep is not what it used to be, most do not feel that poor sleep is significantly interfering with how they feel or function.

If you feel your quality of life is being diminished by sleeping difficulties, do not hesitate to seek help and do not be discouraged by those who would make light of your complaints.

REASONS FOR DISTURBED SLEEP IN OLDER PEOPLE

Sleep Apnea

Sleep apnea is one of several medical conditions that can genuinely interfere with older people's sleep. Sleep apnea has been reported in as many as 30% of the healthy elderly adults who have been studied.[2,3] It probably results from the gradual loss of tone in the muscles in the upper airway, which occurs with increasing age.

The sleep apnea seen in healthy older people is usually very mild or moderate. In many cases it is not severe enough, or is barely severe enough, to qualify as clinical sleep apnea (that is, more than five apnea events of ten seconds or more during an hour, or a total of 30 or more apnea events during a night).[4]

The consensus seems to be that a moderate degree of apnea in otherwise healthy older people does not normally call for treatment. However, a suspicion of sleep apnea should not be ignored. Drowsiness and loss of mental alertness are the worst enemies of the healthy senior citizen, whose goal should be to remain as active and alert as possible. Apnea episodes contribute both to fragmentation of sleep and to a decrease in the oxygen content in the blood, which can lead to daytime drowsiness and loss of alertness. Seniors with other kinds of sleep disturbances, such as restless legs, show less daytime drowsiness.[2] This suggests that sleep apnea may be a particularly important cause of the daytime drowsiness seen in seniors.

If you are an older person who suspects that apnea is significantly disturbing your sleep and is causing drowsiness during the daytime, you may want to contact a sleep center for an interview and potential testing.

Leg Movements During Sleep

Some 40% of older adults experience involuntary leg movements associated with sleep. In *restless legs syndrome*, a person has a tingly feeling and an urge to move the legs. This may interfere with falling asleep. *Periodic leg movements (nocturnal myoclonus)* are kicking motions that occur repeatedly during sleep. These may awaken the sleeper, but often they do not and are more disruptive to the bedpartner. If you or your bedpartner experiences either of these disorders, talk with a sleep specialist about possible treatment.

Medical Problems and Depression

Some less healthy older adults are bothered with medical problems that affect sleep (for example, pain from arthritis and other pain syndromes, respiratory problems, frequent urination, or leg cramps).

Depression is another condition that can affect sleep. The symptoms of depression are often attributed to "just getting old": insomnia; pessimism; loss of interest; decreased energy; poor self-esteem; poor sexual functioning; increase in health complaints, such as constipation, back pain, abdominal pain, headache; social withdrawal; decreased appetite; and weight loss.

However, it is *not* true that getting older inevitably leads to these difficulties. Healthy older adults who are not depressed do not routinely experience these symptoms. If depression is the cause of symptoms such as poor sleep, it is the depression that needs to be treated, not simply the symptoms.

The treatment of medical problems and depression that interfere with sleep is best carried out in consultation with a sleep specialist, as explained later, because some treatments can further interfere with sleep.

GETTING A GOOD NIGHT'S SLEEP

The most common sleep complaint among healthy older people is that they awaken numerous times during the night.[1] Sometimes people become worried about this pattern, and the worry itself—that they're "not getting a good night's sleep"—keeps them awake.

If you are a senior who is bothered somewhat by frequent awakenings during the night and drowsiness during the day and you have ruled out any serious sleep disorder, here are two helpful things that you can do for yourself:

1. Reassure yourself that nighttime awakenings are normal and not something that you need to worry a lot about. You probably are actually getting enough sleep. This knowledge alone may release you from worrying about getting a good night's sleep. That, in turn, will probably let you sleep better.

2. Practice good "sleep hygiene." That is, try arranging your day-time life so that you promote good sleep:
   a. Eat regular meals.
   b. Get more exercise every day (but don't exercise right before bedtime).
   c. Eliminate daytime naps. Often they are more the result of boredom rather than sleepiness. Find something active to do instead of napping.
   d. Plan evening activities—with friends or by yourself, either outside or in the home. Look forward to a full evening.
   e. Limit your caffeine intake (coffee, tea, cocoa, cola) and use alcohol moderately (alcohol actually interferes with sleep).
   f. Limit your fluids after 7 p.m., so that you will have less need to urinate during the night.
   g. Make yourself get out of bed and get dressed at a specif-ic early hour every morning (say, 6:30 or 7).
   h. Learn relaxation techniques to relieve the tension or wor-ries that may be keeping you awake.

If you try these suggestions in a disciplined way for several weeks and decide they are not helpful, make an appointment to discuss the problems with your doctor. If the symptoms are not resolved, ask your doctor about a referral to a sleep clinic.

If you have a medical problem that seems to be interfering with your sleep, check with a sleep specialist for ideas about a solution that will help you sleep better.

Sometimes the treatment for one medical problem may con-flict with the treatment for another. For example, some drugs taken for heart problems can make sleep apnea worse. "Sleeping pills" nearly always make sleep apnea worse, as does alcohol. Barbiturates and some antidepressants have side effects that can affect sleep. A sleep specialist is likely to know more about these effects upon sleep than your family doctor does, and the two of them should work together to find the most appropriate way of improving your night's sleep.

If sleep apnea is a moderate to serious problem for you or if you have other conditions, such as arrhythmias (irregular heart rhythms), congestive heart failure, or respiratory problems, that are aggravated by sleep apnea, the sleep specialist may recommend treatment for your apnea. The type of treatment will depend on the kind of apnea and the severity of the problem. (See Chap. 7 for treatment of sleep apnea.)

Summary

✤ *Older people often get as much total sleep in 24 hours as young people.*

✤ *However, older people's sleep may be of poorer quality; that is, broken up by periods of wakefulness.*

✤ *Factors that can interfere with older people's sleep include sleep apnea, leg movement syndromes, pain, respiratory problems, frequent urination, medications, and depression.*

✤ *Seek help if you are persistently drowsy or if sleep disturbance is decreasing your quality of life.*

✤ *If you suspect sleep apnea, go to an accredited sleep center for an interview and possible testing.*

✤ *Mild sleep problems can often be solved by a program of good "sleep hygiene," discussed in the chapter.*

>>>>> 12 >>>>>

Finding a Sleep Specialist

THE STATE OF THE ART

The field of sleep disorders medicine is a new medical specialty, and the number of doctors who are trained in it is still small.

Most established specialties, such as pediatrics, obstetrics/gynecology, otolaryngology (ear, nose, and throat), psychiatry, and so on, have their own departments in hospitals and medical schools. Medical students are taught courses by specialists in these fields, and they learn routines for diagnosis and treatment of illnesses in those areas. After medical school, doctors can spend several years in residency programs in their chosen specialties, perfecting their skills.

But very few medical schools offer courses or programs in sleep disorders medicine. Consequently, very few doctors are trained to recognize and treat sleep disorders.

In the absence of established departments of sleep medicine in hospitals and medical schools, a number of professional organizations have taken on the role of setting the standards for professionalism in the field. The American Sleep Disorders Association (ASDA), whose members are accredited sleep centers and sleep specialists, has established the standards for the evaluation and treatment of sleep disorders. Its parent organization is the Association of Professional Sleep Societies (APSS), which also includes the Sleep Research Society (SRS). The APSS coordinates the publication of journals dealing with sleep and sponsors conferences on the latest research and treatments for sleep disorders.

These professional organizations today are the backbone of sleep disorders medicine and the main source of learning and information exchange for professionals in the field. In time this will change. The field is growing very rapidly. The American Sleep Disorders Association hopes that within a few years the major medical schools will have programs on sleep disorders. However, until systematic sleep medicine training becomes part of the regular medical school curriculum, the public will have to look carefully to find a qualified sleep specialist.

QUALIFICATIONS OF A SLEEP SPECIALIST

Because so few training programs have existed, most of today's sleep specialists have done their residencies in other, related specialties. In 1991 the ASDA reported the specialties of their members as follows: psychiatrists/neurologists/psychologists (48%), pulmonologists (38%), and other specialties (14%).

These doctors have then gone on to study sleep physiology through additional fellowship programs, graduate courses, or periods of practice at one of the major sleep disorders centers. In 1993 only eight such ASDA-accredited fellowship programs in sleep disorders medicine existed; they were located at Stanford University; Georgetown University Hospital in Washington, DC; Mt. Sinai Medical Center in Miami Beach; VA Medical Center in Allen Park, MI; Henry Ford Hospital in Detroit; University Hospital at Stony Brook, NY; the Medical College of Pennsylvania; and Crozer-Chester Medical Center in Upland, PA.

A physician can earn a sleep specialist credential by passing the certification examination administered by the American Board of Sleep Medicine. He becomes a Board Certified Sleep Specialist (BCSS). (Prior to the recent establishment of this board, the credential for a certified sleep specialist was Accredited Clinical Polysomnographer, or ACP.)

Some physicians who have trained in sleep medicine do not choose to become certified; nevertheless they may be well informed about sleep disorders. However, as in any medical specialty, a doctor's board certificate in sleep medicine assures you, the consumer, that the doctor has received special training and is qualified to carry out sleep testing and to interpret the results of the tests.

You may feel hesitant about asking a doctor about his training and qualifications. But this is especially important in a new field like sleep disorders medicine. "Are you board certified in sleep medicine?" is a perfectly legitimate question. If the doctor appears surprised by your question, you can remind him pleasantly that it is your body he's dealing with. Or find another doctor.

You might also ask your sleep doctor if he is a member of the ASDA. Although membership in a professional group is not mandatory, it indicates something about his involvement in the field and may suggest how well he keeps up with current sleep research.

If you feel reluctant to ask a doctor these questions, call his office and ask his nurse. If she can't answer your questions, ask her to find out and call you back.

Finally, it is not advisable to embark upon a treatment program for a "sleep disorder" before having undergone thorough sleep testing at an accredited sleep disorders clinic. This is particularly true if the treatment involves surgery. Read Chapters 5, 6, and 7, and seek a second opinion.

STANDARDS FOR AN ACCREDITED SLEEP CENTER

An accredited sleep center is one that has met the standards established by the ASDA. As of the summer of 1993 there were more than 250 accredited sleep centers and labs in the United States. In addition, there were more than 1,000 nonaccredited sleep labs nationwide. Some of the nonaccredited sleep labs are very good. However, a very wide range of quality exists, all the way down to some "street corner" sleep labs that are not reputable. The ASDA has neither the funds, the staff, nor the mandate to "police" the entire field of sleep medicine beyond their own membership. And so far no other organization or agency is keeping an eye on the quality of sleep testing that goes on in the non-ASDA-accredited labs.

As a prudent consumer, if you want some assurance of professional standards in this new field, you may want to choose one of the sleep centers accredited by the ASDA.

The standards for accreditation are broken down into two categories: *full-service sleep centers* and *specialty labs*.

Full-Service Sleep Centers

The requirements for accreditation for a full-service sleep center ensure that the center is able to deal professionally with the full range of sleep disorders. Here are the primary ASDA requirements for a full-service sleep center:

❖ It must have an ASDA-accredited clinical polysomnographer (MD or PhD) on staff to read and interpret the results of sleep recordings.

❖ It must have a full-time physician with expertise in sleep physiology.

❖ It must have trained technicians to administer the sleep tests. Sleep centers are encouraged to have at least one technician who is accredited as a Registered Polysomnographic Technologist.

❖ A private room must be provided for each patient, with sound, light, and temperature control and easy communication with the attendant.

❖ The facilities, testing procedures, and patient care must meet standards set by the ASDA.

❖ The sleep center must pass inspection by a two-member accreditation team every five years or lose its accreditation.

Specialty Labs

The standards for accreditation of a specialty lab are similar but tailored to a less extensive sleep testing role. Specialty labs usually deal primarily with pulmonary medicine (breathing disorders), and the diagnostic testing they do is mostly for sleep apnea rather than for the full range of sleep disorders.

The requirements for a specialty lab include the following:

✤ It must have at least one pulmonary specialist on staff.

✤ The staff must demonstrate knowledge of the practices and procedures of sleep disorders medicine.

✤ The physical surroundings, facilities, testing procedures, and patient care must meet ASDA standards similar to those for a full-service sleep center.

HOW TO LOCATE THE NEAREST ACCREDITED SLEEP CENTER

The ASDA will mail you a booklet listing the 250-plus accredited sleep centers in the United States. Write to the ASDA at the following address. Include a long, self-addressed, stamped envelope.

American Sleep Disorders Association
1610 14th Street NW, Suite 300
Rochester, MN 55901-2200

Or call them at (507) 287-6006.

Summary

❖ Certification of sleep spec*ialists and accreditation of sleep centers by the ASDA gives the consumer some assurance of quality.*

❖ *Good noncertified sleep physicians and nonaccredited sleep centers exist. Ask the doctor about his sleep specialty training. Be a prudent consumer.*

❖ *If you want to check the credentials of a sleep specialist or a sleep center, contact the ASDA.*

> > > > > 13 > > > > >

Choosing a CPAP and a Homecare Company

Before you buy a car, you shop around. You may talk to several dealers, compare makes and models, and find out which dealers provide good customer service.

When you need a CPAP (continuous positive airway pressure) machine you may not have time to shop around. Your health is at stake, and you should get started using CPAP as soon as possible after your doctor prescribes it. If you rely on suggestions from your sleep center and from the homecare company they recommend, you will probably be in very good hands.

However, if you do want the luxury of time to shop around, you might consider renting a unit for a time. Shopping can be worthwhile. After all, you will spend more time with your CPAP than you will in your car. The features of that CPAP machine and the homecare service you receive will become important to you.

Case Study (continued). When Mr. Kennedy's sleep specialist prescribed a CPAP machine, Mr. Kennedy had no idea of where to begin. His sleep center recommended that he call a homecare company. He had never heard of homecare companies. He didn't know that he could have chosen between several homecare companies in his area and that different homecare companies may carry different makes and models of CPAP. He didn't know that the features of

CPAP units vary from one manufacturer to another and that he had an option of renting or buying a CPAP.

He called the homecare company that his sleep center recommended and bought the first CPAP he saw. Fortunately, he was content with both decisions. However, if he had it to do over, Mr. Kennedy thinks he would start by renting a CPAP unit. Then he would ask questions about other CPAP models and compare prices and services among several homecare companies. He might try out several masks and CPAP models, on a rental basis, and decide which features are most important to him before buying his own CPAP.

As a CPAP consumer, you have two areas of choice, and options within each area:

1. Homecare provider.
   a. Which homecare companies does your sleep center recommend? Do any have an unfavorable reputation?
   b. What brands and models of CPAP does the homecare company supply?
   c. What are their prices for CPAP units and parts (masks, tubing, filters)?
   d. What services do they include in that price?
2. CPAP.
   a. Quality?
   b. Price?
   c. Unique features (mask fit, size and shape of unit, durability, adaptability, appearance, and so on)?

CHOOSING A HOMECARE COMPANY

If you have never dealt with a homecare company, you may not even be aware of their existence. Homecare companies (sometimes called durable medical equipment, or DME, companies) rent, sell, and service health care equipment for use at home: mechanical ventilators, oxygen, CPAP systems, and other home health care supplies.

Most likely, your first CPAP unit will be delivered to you in your home by a representative of the homecare company you choose. This representative, usually a respiratory therapist, should make sure your CPAP is set up properly and should instruct you about the use of the equipment and answer any questions you have. In-home service to homecare customers is included in the cost of equipment rental or purchase, and 24-hour service should be available when needed.

Here are the names of the largest nationwide homecare companies:

❖ Apria Healthcare Group
❖ Lincare, Inc.

You can find the nearest offices of these and other, more localized homecare companies listed in your Yellow Pages under *Medical Equipment* or *Hospital Equipment and Supplies*. The nationwide homecare companies have branch offices throughout the country, but not all of them may serve your area.

Which homecare company should you choose? Ultimately, the choice of a homecare company is not critical; you can always change companies if you are dissatisfied. But here are some considerations:

1. *Recommendations from others.* Sleep centers usually know which homecare companies offer the best services. Ask the CPAP coordinator or sleep specialist.

Ask other CPAP users. Go to an AWAKE meeting (see Chap. 14 and the Appendix) and find out which homecare companies have given good service to other CPAP users. Or ask your sleep center if they can give you the phone number of a CPAP owner in your community to talk to. You may find that not all branches of a particular homecare company provide equally excellent service. People may tell you that if you live on the north end of town, Company A has the best service, but if you are on the south side, Company B has the best CPAP man.

2. *CPAP brand or model, and the CPAP mask.* Have you decided on a particular CPAP model that you want to use? Which homecare companies handle that brand? Try to choose a homecare company that can service your brand of CPAP adequately.

   Masks vary in size, shape, and fit. A good homecare company will have several brands available for you to try, until you are happy with the fit. Most masks can be used with any model of CPAP machine.

3. *Prices.* Compare prices charged by homecare companies not only for the CPAP unit itself but also for parts and replacements. The mask, headgear, and tubing for your machine will probably be sold separately from the CPAP unit. Replacement of the mask (and for some units the air filter) is necessary periodically.

4. *Service.* Remember that you are paying a homecare company not only for equipment but also for service. What services do they offer automatically? The following is the minimum you should expect from a good homecare company:

   a. Home delivery of your new CPAP unit by a trained homecare representative. The homecare representative should be thoroughly familiar with your model of CPAP. He/she should explain exactly how to use the unit, make sure the pressure setting is correct for you, be certain the mask is the right size and help you adjust the headgear, explain how to clean and care for the equipment, answer any questions you might have, and continue to work closely with you for as long as it takes you to feel you have a comfortable, trouble-free CPAP setup.

   b. Annual servicing of your CPAP unit. You may have to ask for this, and you may have to pay the cost of renting a replacement while your own unit is being serviced.

   c. Prompt and accurate handling of all paperwork and insurance procedures.

   d. Prompt filling of orders (delivery within 48 hours) for new masks, filters, or other replacement parts.

    e. Same-day service for repairs or a "loaner" to use until your unit is repaired.

    f. Twenty-four-hour service in case of emergency.

If you are ever unhappy with the service you receive, do not hesitate to change companies.

CHOOSING A CPAP

To obtain a CPAP unit from a homecare company, you need a doctor's prescription. Insurance companies will not cover the cost of rental or purchase of a CPAP system unless sleep studies have been done to document the medical necessity for CPAP. Talk with your insurance company before obtaining a CPAP, so that you will know in advance which costs they will cover.

Numerous makes and models of CPAP are available. This technology is growing and changing so rapidly that we cannot describe specific makes or models; by the time you read this the information would be out of date. The important thing is to compare features. This is why it may be a good idea to rent and try out a model or two before you purchase. Each model has its unique features, so the choice may seem confusing at first.

CPAP masks are sold separately. The comfort and fit of the mask are very important. Numerous brands and sizes of standard masks are available. There are also some smaller devices that use a pair of little pads that fit up against the nostrils. For infants and children the Bubble Mask™ is reported to work very well. Most of these alternatives can be used with any model of CPAP. Keep trying different masks until you find the one that works best for you.

Let's look at three major areas of comparison among CPAP units: quality, price, and special features.

Quality: Reliability and Performance

You need a CPAP unit with:

1. Reliability. It must work properly all night, every night.

2. Performance. It must be capable of delivering a constant level of air pressure, even when there is a leak around the mask.

In deciding upon a brand, the least risky choice would be one of the top manufacturers. All have established track records for supplying high-quality products, parts, service, and support for their products. At this writing the four leading manufacturers are the following:

❖ ResMed (formerly ResCare)
  5744 Pacific Center Blvd., Suite 311
  San Diego, CA 92121
  619-622-2040

❖ Respironics, Inc.
  1001 Murry Ridge Dr.
  Murrysville, PA 15668
  412-733-0200

❖ Healthdyne
  1255 Kennestone Circle
  Marietta, GA 30066
  404-499-1212

❖ Puritan Bennett
  10800 Pflumm Road
  Lenexa, KA 66215
  913-469-5400

ResMed grew out of Baxter Healthcare, Inc., which in 1986 supported the commercial development of the original CPAP technology invented by Dr. Colin Sullivan in Australia. ResCare/Baxter was the first to incorporate several innovative features into CPAP: the universal power supply (1988); the delay timer, or "ramp" function (1989); and the Bubble Mask™ (1991). ResCare prides itself on being innovative.

Respironics was the first manufacturer to make CPAP units commercially available. They have steadily improved their product while continuing to provide good service. The Respironics CPAP unit is simple in design. The newer versions are beltless and adaptable for AC/DC current as well as European circuits. As mentioned in Chapter 7, the company introduced a system in 1990 called BiPAP™, with two variable-pressure settings.

Healthdyne and Puritan Bennett both have fine CPAP units on the market. Both companies have manufactured other types of hospital equipment for many years and are large firms with solid track records.

All these manufacturers have regional or local representatives who visit the sleep centers and the homecare companies that carry their brand and train the employees in the proper use and maintenance of the equipment.

Price

At this writing, CPAP rentals are about $200 per month, and the purchase price is in the neighborhood of $1,200. You may have to purchase the mask and tubing separately (about $130 total). (These prices may vary across the country.) The mask material tends to absorb oil from the skin and to become stiff, needing to be replaced about every six months, so that is a recurring expense. Some models have nonwashable air filters that need periodic replacement.

Compare the prices for a particular model among several local homecare companies. Ask what additional equipment and services they provide for that price. Find out what costs your insurance company will cover.

Special Features

Your *CPAP mask* must fit securely and comfortably. Getting the mask to fit properly is probably the biggest frustration most people encounter with CPAP. Most people find they need to experiment with the mask for a while to get a comfortable, leak-free fit. (See Chapter 15 for suggestions on mask fit.) Having a mask that is the right size is important. Your homecare representative should be willing to try different sizes and brands of mask until you have an acceptable fit. If you experience leaks, chafing, or other problems, ask for more help from your homecare company. Ask about trying a Bubble Mask™, or try one of the "nasal pad" alternatives. Some people find these more comfortable than the mask; others do not. Experiment. Don't give up!

Each model of CPAP advertises individual features that make it unique. Your particular lifestyle, taste, or leisure activities may make one model more appealing to you than another.

You may also want to give some thought to future activities— things you would enjoy doing once you have more energy. It is common for CPAP users to discover that soon they are able to be more active than they had been when they were slowed down by sleepiness or poor health. What would *you* like to do when you feel better? Take a trip to Europe; invite your sweetie to spend the night; go car camping, backpacking, or traveling across the country in an RV; charter a sailboat...? What features in a CPAP would enable you to fulfill that wish?

Size or shape might be important to you. Does the CPAP unit need to fit on your nightstand, or can it just sit on the floor? If you travel a lot, will it be easy to carry? Prudent CPAP travelers carry their units onto planes, rather than checking them through as baggage, to avoid the risk of loss or damage. Most CPAPs will fit into a carry-on bag and slide easily under an airplane seat. The slimmest new models might even fit in a briefcase. Some manufacturers offer an attractive *carrying case* that is probably roomy enough to also hold a woman traveler's nightgown and cosmetics.

If you travel, does the unit seem *durable* and sturdy enough to stand up to the stress?

How about *electrical adaptability*? U.S. electrical circuits operate at 110 volts and 60 Hz (cycles per second). Many European countries use 220 to 240 volts and 50 Hz. If you travel outside the United States, find out which CPAP models can be plugged into or readily adapted for European circuits. One manufacturer (ResCare) even has a unit that has been approved for use on a Boeing 747 (110 V, 400 Hz). If you are a car camper or boater or if you have a recreational vehicle, what electric source will you want to use, and how easily can your CPAP be adapted? Many active CPAP users are looking forward to the advent of more battery-friendly models. One avid backpacker is lobbying for a mini-CPAP machine that could run on solar batteries attached to his hat! Who can even imagine the wonders that technology may bring?

Are you or your bedpartner sensitive to noises during sleep? Listen to the CPAP's *sound*. Most CPAPs nowadays are so quiet that they produce only a gentle "white noise," which some people find actually lulls them to sleep. Test the sound with the unit turned on and while wearing the mask and breathing normally. Listen to the sound of the machine and the escaping air.

Is the *appearance* of the CPAP important to you? Do you care what it looks like sitting on your bedside table? One model is tastefully designed to look like an air filter unit. Another model permits a book or a cup to be placed on top.

Some people find that their nasal passages become stuffy or dry when using CPAP. A *humidifier* can help alleviate these problems. Some CPAP models have a built-in humidifier, one of which is heated. You may want to ask about these.

Some CPAPs have a *"ramp"* feature, which starts the machine at a low air pressure and increases it slowly over a period of 30 to 45 minutes. Many people find that this gradual increase in air pressure allows them to go to sleep more easily.

The staff of your sleep center have extensive experience with a variety of CPAP units. They may have several makes and models that you can examine. You may want to ask them which manufacturer they prefer. Sleep centers usually choose manufacturers that they consider reliable suppliers of equipment and parts. Their choice may be a good recommendation.

Finally, as mentioned earlier, a homecare company may deal with only one or two CPAP manufacturers, so you may end up choosing the CPAP that your favorite homecare company supplies. Or, conversely, you may choose the homecare company that supplies the brand of CPAP you want.

Summary

❖ Ask your insurance company which CPAP costs it will cover (purchase, rental, parts, service).

❖ Consider renting a CPAP while you shop for a homecare company and the CPAP model of your choice.

❖ When choosing a homecare company, compare local reputation, the brands of CPAP they sell, prices, and services.

❖ When choosing a CPAP, consider quality, price, recommendations from a sleep center, and unique features, such as size, shape, durability, adaptability, appearance, sound, and availability of ramp setting and humidifier

>>>>> 14 >>>>>

Follow-up Care: Living with Sleep Apnea

Everyone with sleep apnea shares the hope that someday this disorder can be cured and forgotten. Today, unfortunately, no sure cure exists, and treatment with CPAP remains the best alternative for most people.

A few lucky people are exceptions, of course. Occasionally, excess weight is the main cause of the sleep apnea, and if the extra weight is lost and kept off, the sleep apnea is held at bay. And for some people surgery eliminates sleep apnea. However, even these fortunate individuals may find that, with increasing age, the sleep apnea symptoms will reappear and will again require medical attention.

For most people sleep apnea is a long-term proposition. Treatment must be continued on a regular basis to stay healthy.

For this reason it is important for people with sleep apnea to receive good follow-up care from their health care providers. Follow-up care affects more than just health. Nearly every aspect of a person's life may be touched by the quality of the continuing care he receives: his image of himself, his family relationships, his sexual life, his vitality and enjoyment of social and leisure activities, his work performance, his career—indeed, his life expectancy.

FOLLOW-UP CARE DETERMINES YOUR FUTURE GOOD HEALTH

The key to effective treatment of any medical disorder is a question of *compliance*: does the person use the treatment, and use it consistently?

Surveys have shown that, for CPAP, the cornerstone of compliance is *follow-up care*: is the person receiving the kind of support he needs to be able to comply with the treatment? As one health care team has stated, "The most brilliant sleep diagnosis is meaningless if the plan for treatment is misunderstood or if the patient is non-compliant. Sleep specialists have a commitment to the patient to go beyond diagnosis."[1]

If a person with sleep apnea is simply handed a CPAP machine and told to go home and use it, the chances of his continuing the treatment are very poor. On the other hand, in sleep centers whose follow-up care is thoughtful and thorough, more than eight out of ten CPAP users will continue to use the equipment faithfully and successfully every night.

GETTING THE CARE YOU NEED

Let's assume your doctor has prescribed CPAP, since that is the most common treatment for sleep apnea. You will probably find that the recipe for trouble-free treatment involves two main ingredients:

1. Problem solving and perseverance with CPAP. (We will discuss CPAP problem solving in detail in Chap. 15.)
2. A team effort.

Your Team

You should consider the following people to be members of the team that is dedicated to helping you get on with life:

❖ Your spouse or partner.
❖ Other family members.
❖ The sleep specialist.
❖ The sleep center staff.

❖ The family physician (perhaps).
❖ The representative of the homecare company that supplies the CPAP equipment.
❖ AWAKE, the patient support group.
❖ You—the person being treated for sleep apnea.

Friends and Family

How are friends and family involved in follow-up care? Close friends and family members are very important sources of support. It is good for them to be included in the treatment process so that they can be interested and well informed about CPAP from the beginning. If friends and family are enthusiastic about the results of the treatment and can be encouraging and tolerant during the frustrating but temporary adjustment period, then the person with sleep apnea will feel happier about using CPAP on a regular basis.

Your bedpartner and family may take awhile to get used to having CPAP around the house and to the notion that you need to use it when you sleep. It may help if everyone thinks of CPAP as they would a pair of glasses. The first person who ever wore eyeglasses probably looked fairly peculiar—but it must have been worthwhile to see better, and soon people got used to the idea. CPAP is like a pair of glasses: a device that solves a problem and enhances life. With that outlook CPAP may seem less like a weird piece of medical equipment and you may feel less like an "invalid" and more like someone who just happens to have sleep apnea.

Your team includes two important groups of professionals: sleep center staff and homecare companies. Let's look at how they can contribute to your continuing care.

The Sleep Center's Role in Follow-up Care

The Ideal Follow-up

Your sleep specialist who prescribes your sleep apnea treatment will probably emphasize the importance of sticking with the treatment. After that, it will be up to members of the sleep center staff and the homecare company to work with you from then on, making sure you are able to carry out the prescription.

Some sleep centers have a staff member who acts as CPAP contact person, takes care of follow-up, arranges appointments with nutritionists, counselors, and other specialists, and generally makes sure that people's questions get answered and problems get solved. Often this is a nurse specialist, a nurse practitioner, a sleep technician, or some other well trained paramedical person.

The trained staff person should be available to make sure that the treatment, be it a weight loss program or a CPAP unit, is tailored to your individual needs. The staff should remain available to you and your family to answer questions and help solve any problems that may arise in the future.

The ideal solution is found at sleep centers that have an actual follow-up clinic to which all patients are referred, whether

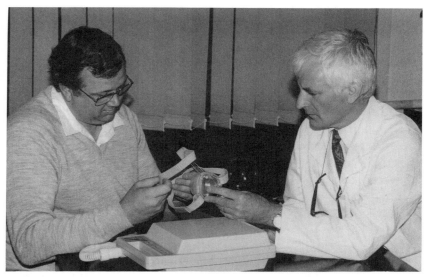

FIG. 14.1. A CPAP user consults with a sleep center staff member about the use of his machine.

they are being treated by the sleep center or by an outside physician. The follow-up clinic offers self-help meetings for people with sleep disorders and their families, monitors the progress of treatment, refers people for nutritional counseling, supervised exercise programs, psychological counseling, and other services as needed. This type of comprehensive follow-up for sleep apnea is becoming more common as sleep centers become better established and able to provide more staff services.

Problems with Sleep Centers

In some cases follow-up care is not what it should be, for a number of reasons. First of all, sleep disorder treatment is a new field and is still in a period of rapid change. Some small sleep labs may do only sleep testing and may pass along the treatment and follow-up care to a family physician, who may have little experience with sleep apnea and little time to do adequate follow-up.

Most sleep centers are extremely busy, and some simply do not have enough staff to do complete follow-up with every patient. They are torn between the demand to diagnose new patients, many of whose health is seriously jeopardized by untreated sleep disorders, and the need to keep up with the growing backlog of people under treatment who need continuing care.

You, the patient, are caught in the middle. As always, the key is to ask for help—and to keep asking.

If you can get in touch with an AWAKE group, the nationwide patient support network (discussed later), you may find that other people with sleep apnea can help you. They are especially resourceful in solving CPAP equipment problems.

Homecare Companies

What to Expect

Your homecare representative should be your chief CPAP equipment problem solver. Typically, this relationship begins when the homecare company representative delivers your first CPAP unit to your home. (See Chap. 13 for a list of other services to expect from a homecare company.)

Homecare representatives often are respiratory therapists and have been trained by the manufacturer of the CPAP equipment. They should understand the features and the operation of the equipment and should make sure that the mask and headgear fit you properly.

As you begin to use your CPAP, if you continue to have leaks around the mask, discomfort, or other difficulties, call your homecare representative right away. A persistently badly fitting mask can be so discouraging that you may feel tempted to give up on CPAP altogether. Don't! Call your homecare representative *before* you reach that extreme. He should be available to work with you until you are happy with the results. That is the business of a homecare company, and you are paying for the service.

In case of an actual equipment breakdown, you can call your homecare company anytime, night or day. A broken CPAP results in a breathless, sleepless, stressful night and is a major inconvenience. Veteran CPAP users recall that the fan belts in the old models had a way of failing the night before a crucial meeting or during an important business trip. A good homecare company would deliver a new fan belt at 2 a.m. if a patient needed one. You should expect nothing less than prompt, dependable, 24-hour emergency service from your homecare company. If they cannot give you same-day service for repairs, they should provide a "loaner" CPAP for you to use until your unit is repaired.

CPAP equipment breakdowns are rare, but don't wait for one to happen. If you suspect your CPAP is developing a problem, have your homecare company check it over immediately. Also, have them test the pressure once or twice a year. Some CPAP manufacturers recommend an annual maintenance checkup.

Problems with Homecare Companies

Homecare companies, like other service-oriented businesses, vary in their quality and diligence.

The homecare respiratory therapists who come out to the home are generally sympathetic and helpful. But there seems to be a fairly high turnover rate. Consequently, service may vary. The therapist may or may not be familiar with a particular model of CPAP equipment. He may or may not know how to answer pertinent questions or solve complex problems that may arise.

In addition, communication between sleep centers and homecare companies may be incomplete. For example, homecare representatives typically know very little about sleep disorders or how they affect the patient. They may never have visited a sleep lab and may have no idea what a patient has experienced in undergoing a sleep test. Conversely, your sleep center may not be familiar with the capabilities, limitations, and service records of all the homecare companies in your region.

Consequently, you, the client, are the communication device that sits between the sleep center and the homecare company. You are in a position to educate the homecare people about sleep apnea and its effects on your life. If their service does not meet your needs, explain and complain. If you are dissatisfied, change homecare companies.

You can also educate the sleep center about which homecare companies are doing their jobs well and which are not. Sleep centers can use this information to encourage better service and to steer other patients.

In summary, remember that when you buy or rent a CPAP from a homecare company, part of what you pay for is "service," and you should expect that service to be good. If your homecare company will not satisfy your needs, find another one.

AWAKE: Your Support Group

Other people with sleep apnea can play an enormously helpful role in your follow-up care. Some sleep centers encourage regular meetings of sleep apnea people and their families, both before and after treatment. Individuals have a chance to meet others who have faced the same worries and solved the same problems with which they themselves are grappling. Support groups like these are extremely reassuring and resourceful.

There is a nationwide network of sleep apnea support groups called AWAKE (Alert, Well, And Keeping Energetic). AWAKE groups operate in conjunction with an existing sleep center. Usually the clinic staff launches the group, with the participation of a core of interested people with sleep apnea. From then on the members operate the group, with support from the sleep clinic staff and sometimes from representatives of homecare companies. Some groups meet monthly; others, less frequently.

The purpose of AWAKE groups is to give people with sleep apnea an opportunity for both support and learning. They share their experiences, problems, solutions, and successes with each other, and they exchange information. Some groups publish newsletters. Many invite speakers to their meetings: doctors, homecare representatives, CPAP manufacturers' representatives, and so on.

By the summer of 1993 there were over 100 AWAKE groups throughout the country, with more being started all the time.

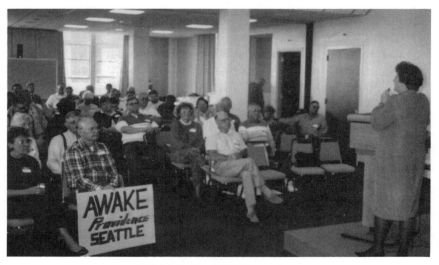

FIG.14.2. An AWAKE meeting.

Ask your local sleep center or homecare company for the location of the nearest AWAKE group. By all means try to attend a meeting. If there is no AWAKE group near you, with the cooperation of your sleep clinic you may be able to help start one. Don't be in the position of sitting at home, reinventing the wheel, when you could so easily be helped by the combined experiences of dozens of other people just like yourself who have found creative solutions that they are eager to share. And you, in turn, will have the pleasure of helping other people by sharing your own insights and answers.

AWAKE is affiliated with another source of patient support, the American Sleep Apnea Association (ASAA), a national dues-for-membership organization for people with sleep apnea and their families and friends. This organization, founded in 1992, is dedicated to public education and fundraising for research on sleep apnea. Members receive an interesting quarterly newsletter.

The addresses of the national AWAKE Network office and the ASAA are in the Appendix.

YOU: THE CAPTAIN OF YOUR TEAM

You are the most important member of your treatment team! You are responsible for your health: for choosing, using, cleaning, and caring for your CPAP equipment. If you have unsolved treatment problems, ultimately the best solution is for you to be utterly relentless. Don't give up! Ask questions until you get answers. You *can* find answers if you are persistent. Read Chapter 15 on CPAP problem solving, and start trying alternatives. If you still have a problem, get in touch with the sleep specialist who first evaluated you. If he is difficult to reach or can't help, ask him to refer you to someone who can. Keep asking. Every problem has a solution. You can find it.

Summary

✤ *Sleep centers and homecare companies have an obligation to provide adequate follow-up care.*

✤ *If you have follow-up questions or problems, assert yourself until your needs are met, or find another sleep center or homecare company.*

✤ *AWAKE is an excellent nationwide patient support organization for people with sleep apnea. Local chapters have scheduled meetings. To locate the closest AWAKE chapter, contact your sleep center, homecare company, or call the AWAKE Network*

>>>>> 15 >>>>>

Solving CPAP Problems

CPAP promises a renewal of life. Until a few years ago, people with sleep apnea had a choice between drowsiness, illness, and probable early death, or a permanent tracheostomy. Today, like butterflies from cocoons, CPAP users can emerge from their private twilight, spread their wings, recapture their health, and rekindle their lives.

Problem solved. Right? Well, no. Unfortunately, adjusting to CPAP sometimes is not quite that easy.

If we were to listen in on an AWAKE group, the magnitude of the adjustment to CPAP would be obvious from the conversation. New CPAP users invariably are concerned with basic problems: mask leaks, stuffy nose, irritated skin, dry mouth. However, we would also hear proof that these problems can be solved. Experienced CPAP users' interests move on to other topics: the newest CPAP models, the latest gimmicks for camping with CPAP, the lack of public awareness about sleep apnea.

Nearly everyone runs into similar adjustments and frustrations when they begin using CPAP. Typically, the questions and problems fall into four general areas:

1. CPAP equipment: troubleshooting.
2. Mental adjustments.
3. Compliance: factors affecting use/nonuse of the equipment.
4. Treatment effectiveness: extent of "cure" and need for re-testing.

Let's look at these one at a time.

187

CPAP EQUIPMENT: TROUBLESHOOTING

We will assume that, if CPAP has been prescribed, you have already had a chance to try CPAP during a night in the sleep center. In most sleep centers if a person is suspected of having sleep apnea, he will be introduced to CPAP equipment while he is being prepared for his sleep test. The technician explains how CPAP works, and eventually the person has a chance to sleep with the device during the night in the sleep lab. This allows the sleep technician to custom-set the CPAP pressure for this particular individual, a process called *titration*. Titration of the CPAP pressure is very important: your CPAP pressure must be high enough to eliminate your sleep apnea, but it should be no higher than necessary, to avoid causing you unnecessary discomfort.

So you have tried CPAP and are ready begin using it at home. Your first unit is likely to be either rented or purchased from a homecare company. (See Chap. 13 on choosing a CPAP unit and a homecare company.)

Patience and Persistence Pay

Every new CPAP user goes through a period of adjustment, becoming familiar with using the equipment, becoming accustomed to wearing the mask, sleeping with it on, and keeping it clean. You, as a new CPAP user, will go through this adjustment period. Some people get used to CPAP in a couple of nights and never have a single problem. Most run into some frustrations. The most common frustrations are difficulty with the fit of the mask and the headgear, leakage problems, stuffy nose, and dry throat. Also, some people take a while to get used to the sound of the motor running during the night or of air escaping through the valve or vents.

All these adjustments are temporary, but can be annoying. They require *perseverance* on the part of the CPAP user and his family: perseverance until the person feels comfortable enough with the CPAP equipment and enthusiastic enough about its effectiveness that he is willing to continue to use it every night.

The key is to ask questions. Don't give up. Turn to the people on your team (see Chap. 14) for assistance as soon as you run into a problem. Seek advice from the professionals: the sleep center staff, the homecare representative from whom you obtained your CPAP machine. And feel free to talk to other CPAP users, through the AWAKE network (see Appendix). These people have solutions to your problems.

Mask Fit and Leakage Problems

Air leakage around the mask and chafing of the bridge of the nose are two of the most common problems with CPAP. The reasons usually are *the mask is the wrong size or shape* or *the headgear is too tight or unevenly adjusted.*

By testing the fit of several masks and fiddling with the adjustments, you will eventually hit upon the right combination. Most masks come in several sizes, and each brand has a slightly different shape and fit. Ask your homecare representative to bring you a selection of mask sizes and brands, and to sit down with you and help you adjust the headgear. Try on the masks with your CPAP machine running.

A common reason for chafing on the bridge of the nose is overtightening the headgear. If your mask fits properly, you shouldn't have to tighten the headgear to the point of chafing. Try wearing it a little *looser* or adding a *spacer* at the top.

A Bubble Mask™ may solve your leakage problems. This mask is made from a thin membrane material that forms a "rolling seal" against the face. It uses much looser headgear and has a softer fit that generally eliminates chafing problems. Bubble Masks™ can be used with any CPAP system.

If you still have a leak, another trick you might try is to put a soft, cushiony material between the mask and your skin. This also works for people whose skin is allergic to the mask material. Microfoam tape (from the 3M Company; ask your homecare representative) can be taped to the mask. Or you might try using a "go-between": a shield to keep the mask from touching the skin. To make a go-between, cut a 4- or 5-inch square (a little larger than the footprint of the mask) out of soft, white fabric, such as felt or thin terrycloth, and then cut a big triangle out of the middle for your nose to fit through. Place the fabric between the mask and your face.

There have been rare cases of eye irritation or infection either caused or aggravated by air escaping from around a poorly fitting mask. In case of eye irritation notify your sleep specialist. CPAP will probably have to be discontinued until the irritation clears up.

A *worn-out mask* will fit poorly and cause chafing. A silicone mask should last for 12 to 18 months, depending on the oiliness of your skin and on how careful you are about cleanliness. Skin oil causes the mask material to become stiff. Order a new mask as soon as the old one starts chafing or fitting poorly. Wearing an ill-fitting mask results in leaks and in skin abrasions that are difficult to heal.

Cleanliness of both mask and skin is extremely important. Washing your face every night before putting on the CPAP will help prevent both skin irritations and mask breakdown. If you have very oily skin, you may want to use a mild astringent, such as witch hazel, around the nose area. To extend the life of your mask the most important thing you can do is to wash it with a mild, fragrance-free soap as soon as you take it off in the morning. Overdrying the mask by running the motor with the mask on the end of the hose may also dry it out. Let the mask air-dry.

Once you have a sore spot on the bridge of your nose, healing may be difficult because the mask will tend to irritate it every night. To *prevent abrasion* of the bridge of the nose and/or promote healing, look for wound-care products like Restore™ or Duoderm™. Ask your homecare company. Or try Second Skin™, a blister remedy that you can find in stores that sell running shoes or sports equipment.

A couple of alternatives to the mask use small, soft nasal "pillows" or pads that fit right up against the nostrils. The arrangement is somewhat less cumbersome than the mask, and can be used with any standard CPAP machine. Some people prefer this alternative; others try it but don't like it, and go back to their mask. If you are curious, ask your homecare company or sleep center if they have a set of nasal pads for you to try out.

Dry Mouth

Some people find that their mouth dries out during the night wearing CPAP. This usually results from sleeping with the mouth open. If dry mouth is a problem for you, you may want to try using a *chin strap* to help keep your mouth closed. Keeping a glass of water by the bedside is also a good idea.

Nasal Congestion or Dryness

If you encounter congestion, sneezing, or dry nose, you might want to try using a humidifier. A number of CPAP units come with a humidifier. A special, heated humidifier has recently been introduced that can be used with all makes of CPAP machine, including older units. One manufacturer (ResCare) offers a disposable, mask-insert humidifier that they claim is very effective and works for up to two weeks. Ask your homecare company which humidifiers they recommend.

If your congestion becomes long-term or is caused by allergies, ask your sleep specialist to recommend a decongestant. Some are better for people with sleep apnea than others.

Claustrophobia and Mask Removal

Some people have trouble keeping the CPAP mask on all night. They may have a feeling of claustrophobia, or they may unconsciously pull the mask off during sleep. If you are having either of these difficulties, contact your sleep specialist and discuss the matter with him. These problems can be temporary: there are ways of working through them, so that you can reach a point of being able to sleep quietly without being bothered by CPAP. The benefits you will receive from nightly use of CPAP are definitely worth the effort.

Noise

The newer CPAPs are so much quieter than the vacuum-cleaner-like earlier versions that noise almost isn't an issue anymore.

If noise is a problem for you or your bedpartner, there are many creative options. An obvious one is *earplugs*. Try the kind shaped like soft, foam cylinders. They are quite comfortable. If you have had your CPAP sitting next to you on the floor or on a night stand, try *moving your CPAP* to the foot of your bed. If your bedroom closet is roomy and has good air circulation, you can run your CPAP unit there. Leave the door open several inches to let air in. With long enough tubing, you can even run the CPAP from the hall or an adjacent room. One ingenious CPAP user bracketed the machine to the ceiling of the room below the bedroom, and ran the tubing up through a hole. These are the kinds of creative solutions you will hear about at AWAKE meetings, from people who have been there.

MENTAL ADJUSTMENTS

Mental adjustments are also part of getting used to CPAP. As a new CPAP user, you will have to become accustomed to seeing yourself as someone who needs this rather unusual piece of equipment in order to maintain good health. Some people—particularly young people in their 40s with sleep apnea—may understandably have difficulty accepting the image of themselves as people with a chronic medical condition.

It is natural to wonder how this whole treatment process is going to affect relationships with friends and other members of the family. Will your kids think you are an invalid? And what about your sex life? Will your wife/husband still find you attractive? What will your new lover think about that CPAP on your night stand?

> **Case Study**. Mrs. Carter worried the first time she spent the night in the home of friends. What would they think? Would the sound of the CPAP disturb the baby sleeping in the next room? On her first business trip after starting to use her CPAP, she felt self-conscious around her associates and wondered what they thought about her carrying her CPAP onto the plane.

For months Mrs. Carter scurried around feeling as if she had to conceal the fact that she had a sleep disorder and required the use of an unusual piece of medical equipment.

In time, she began tentatively to talk with friends and associates about sleep apnea, and found that they were interested, curious to learn more, and very supportive. She even began to feel good about educating people, and realized that she had become a kind of ambassador for sleep apnea.

"Eventually," Mrs. Carter says, "you simply reach a point of accepting yourself as a person who has sleep apnea and uses a CPAP. Period. And you get on with life."

Depression is an unexpected but fairly common result after sleep apnea is successfully treated, and it demands effective follow-up attention.

Why would a person become depressed after successful treatment? This can happen when a person undergoes a big change, in a very short time, from sleepy and sedentary to awake and active. Following successful treatment, former sleepy people may be pushed abruptly into the active life surrounding them. Friends and family may suddenly interact with them more and expect more of them, and they may doubt their own ability to perform. Family conflicts and feelings of social inadequacy may arise. The former patient may feel at a loss about how to deal with this change.

Another common reaction is one of bitterness over having lost a number of good years of one's life. Many sleep apnea people have spent their prime midlife years in a state of deep somnolence. When they "awaken" after treatment, they feel resentment and loss at having been robbed of those good years. People may need to allow themselves some time to grieve before they can let go of those years and get on with life.

Other adjustments occur in the workplace. After treatment a former sleep apnea patient often is literally a different person from the lethargic, sleepy person his colleagues had become accustomed to. It may take him awhile to retrain those coworkers to recognize the "new" person's capabilities. If you find yourself in this frustrating situation, it may help just to remember to allow both yourself and your colleagues some time to adjust.

The spouse or partner of someone who has been treated for sleep apnea also has some adjustments to make. She has become accustomed to life with a sleepy person. Perhaps she has had to take over a lot of the family, household, and financial tasks and now must learn to share them again. If her spouse has been very sick, she may even have prepared herself emotionally for his death. The transformation of her partner into someone with unexpected vitality and energy may be a shock. She may not at once welcome such an abrupt change. She may be surprised to feel a confusing mixture of emotions, from anxiety to resentment to guilt.

These are all very significant adjustments, and most people with sleep apnea have to deal with some of them. If you attend an AWAKE meeting (see Chap. 14), you will discover that you are not alone in having adjustments to make. It may help to talk with others who have been through similar experiences. Counseling can also be helpful, for the individual or the whole family, giving people a chance to talk over their concerns. Your sleep specialist or the sleep center staff can recommend a counselor.

THE IMPORTANCE OF COMPLIANCE

People fail to comply with CPAP for many reasons. As mentioned earlier, the root cause of noncompliance usually is inadequate follow-up care: either the CPAP user has not been properly introduced to CPAP, he does not receive proper follow-up help, or he does not understand what sleep apnea will do to his health if he does not use his CPAP regularly.

You should understand that CPAP is literally a lifesaver for you. You need to use CPAP *every time you go to sleep*—even for naps, even when you spend just one overnight away from home. Use CPAP because it offers you better health and longer life than you can expect if your sleep apnea is not treated. CPAP is your ticket to enjoying the things in life that are most important to you—instead of giving in to sleepiness, exhaustion, and poor health.

If your sleep center does not automatically offer the degree of continuing care you need, *do not hesitate to request additional attention.* You should receive whatever assistance you need to continue your CPAP treatment.

Again the key is to ask for help. If you are having an equipment problem, as mentioned earlier, sleep center and homecare staff can help you with troubleshooting. Other patients, contacted through AWAKE, can be enormously helpful, because they have been there and can understand what you are dealing with. There is no problem that cannot be worked out. Solve the problem, so that you can continue with the treatment and get on with your life. A CPAP unit does nobody any good if it spends the night unplugged in the closet.

TREATMENT EFFECTIVENESS

"I feel cured. Can I stop using CPAP?" Probably not. It is very common for people to report dramatic results from treatment. In fact, they often feel more improvement than has actually occurred. After UPPP surgery, a person may feel "completely cured," only to discover, after retesting, that he still has 50% of his sleep apnea. So don't assume, just because you feel better, that your sleep apnea has necessarily been thoroughly treated. And, most important, don't assume that, because you feel better, you can stop treatment. If you stop treatment, your sleep apnea will come back.

Sleep apnea patients usually are asked to return to the sleep center after a specified period of treatment to be retested to verify that the treatment is effective. This is true not only for CPAP users but also for sleep apnea patients who are being treated with medication, and those who have undergone surgery.

Another reason to be retested is if your treatment has *not* given you as much improvement as you had expected. Occasionally a patient returns for retesting and the technicians find that the pressure on his CPAP unit was not set properly. Or the sleep specialist discovers a second sleep disorder that was missed during the initial sleep test. So if you think you should be feeling better than you are, contact your sleep specialist.

Periodic retesting is important for all patients, over the years, to make sure that the treatment remains effective and that there is no return of the symptoms of sleep apnea. Most sleep centers will tell you when they want you to return for retesting. If yours does not tell you, ask.

ON BEING A PIONEER

Today's sleep apnea people are medical pioneers. You are helping to teach the medical community how to recognize and treat sleep apnea. You are helping the sleep disorder centers to learn how to meet their patients' needs. You are helping the medical researchers and medical equipment manufacturers to invent better treatment methods.

The sleep disorders field is young, and it still has some weaknesses. The understanding of sleep apnea throughout the medical community is not yet widespread. But there are many well-informed doctors, many excellent sleep specialists, and many superb sleep centers in the United States and throughout the world.

And, most important, today there are simple, effective treatments for sleep apnea that didn't exist two years ago. There is hope now for many people who previously could not expect to see their sixtieth birthday.

You and your partner need to be assertive, well-informed consumers in this new field. Make sure your needs are met, because in a new field it's a little bit harder than it should be to get things done. Be patient, but not too patient. Be stubborn. Don't give up! Make sure your doctor listens to you. Seek out the best-equipped, best-staffed sleep centers. Ask questions until you get answers. Learn the treatment options. Choose the conservative treatment over the risky one. Seek second opinions on surgery. Find the experienced surgeons. Keep after your insurance company until they pay for your care. Demand service from your homecare provider, or switch to a competing company. Let them know if you are dissatisfied. And demand adequate follow-up care. It's your life.

CPAP Problems and Who to Call for Help

	Sleep Specialist	Sleep Center Staff	Homecare Company	AWAKE Group
Equipment Problems				
Mask fit, other problems, day-to-day use	Solutions to medical problems: (allergy, infection, inflammation, medications)	Advice, suggestions, troubleshooting	Choice of models, sizes; advice	Advice, suggestions, troubleshooting
Breakdown, repairs			24-hour service	
New products, updates		Advice, information	New equipment	Advice, information
Compliance and Mental Adjustment				
Use/nonuse of CPAP	Discuss problems Encourage Refer for counseling	Problem solving: mask fit, skin irritation	Mask fit, mask leaks, mask size, type, humidifier, service	Encouragement, support, education, problem solving
Treatment Effectiveness				
	Schedule retest	Discuss need for retest		

Summary

✤ *Expect to go through a temporary adjustment period as you get used to using CPAP.*

✤ *Patience, persistence, trial and error, asking questions, and demanding service are the keys to solving CPAP equipment problems.*

➤ ➤ ➤ ➤ ➤ 16 ➤ ➤ ➤ ➤ ➤

Alternative Medicine and Sleep Apnea

C *ase Study.* *Mr. Chambers was having trouble getting used to his CPAP machine. He was still waking up many times during the night, and still feeling fatigued during the day. His sleep center scheduled him for a trial on BiPAP™. With BiPAP™ he slept through the night and felt refreshed the next morning. He arranged to buy a BiPAP unit, and began using it nightly.*

At about the same time, Mr. Chambers read an article promoting magnetism as a treatment for a number of medical complaints, including fatigue. The article described several patients' miraculous cures and claimed that these anecdotes "proved" the effectiveness of magnetism. The author of the article offered several magnetic products for sale.

Mr. Chambers wanted to feel better. He was impressed by the testimonials of the patients who had tried magnetism. He ordered several hundred dollars' worth of magnetic bracelets, magnetic shoe inserts, and magnets to put in his mattress and pillow.

Today Mr. Chambers feels more alert and energetic than ever before. He is convinced that magnetism has revitalized him.

A new field of medicine offers fertile ground for quackery. Unscrupulous people are quick to exploit people's hopes and fears. Claims of miracle cures for sleep apnea are already germinating among the "alternative" medical practitioners.

WHO CAN DIAGNOSE SLEEP APNEA?

Let's be clear on this. For an accurate diagnosis of sleep apnea, you need an overnight sleep test that follows standardized procedures. The results should be evaluated, and the treatment prescribed, by a well-trained, preferably accredited, sleep specialist.

Any alert doctor may suspect sleep apnea by looking at you, asking you if you snore, and performing a physical examination. But for an exact diagnosis and appropriate treatment, you need a sleep test.

CAN "ALTERNATIVE MEDICINE" TREAT OR CURE SLEEP APNEA?

"Alternative medicine" cannot treat or cure sleep apnea. There is no *sure cure* yet for sleep apnea. There is effective *treatment*, but if the treatment is stopped, the sleep apnea will return.

Sleep apnea is a complicated disorder, and the choice of the correct treatment depends on many factors, as explained in Chapter 7. The only known effective treatments for sleep apnea include one or more of the following:

1. CPAP.
2. Weight loss, *for some people.*
3. Certain medications, *for some people.*
4. Certain surgeries, *for some people.*
5. A dental appliance, *for some people.*

QUACK DETECTION: RULES OF THUMB

Quacks are experts at appealing to our natural desire for a swift cure. Mr. Chambers, like most people with sleep apnea, didn't want to sleep with a CPAP machine. He was disappointed that his initial CPAP treatment hadn't worked as well as he had expected. He wanted a simple answer. He fell prey to a quack.

How can you recognize a quack? Whom can you believe? And does it really matter if, like Mr. Chambers, you seem to feel better?

Yes, it does matter, for two practical reasons:

1. *Quackery is expensive.* If you are on a limited budget, you can ill afford to spend your income on quack remedies.
2. *Quackery can kill you,* either directly, with a dangerous product, or indirectly, by failing to treat a fatal disorder properly.

If you want to avoid the expense and risks of quackery, here are some rules of thumb:

1. *Be skeptical.* Question anything that seems too good to be true.
2. *Ask for credentials.* What are the credentials of the person making the claims? Can he document any special training that qualifies him to dispense medical advice?
3. *Follow the money.* Who profits if you spend your money on this product or service? Is the cost reasonable, or is someone offering you a dime-store item for $50?
4. *Question the research.* This is hard to do if you are not a scientist. Good scientific research follows *scientific method.*

HOW DOES SCIENTIFIC METHOD WORK IN MEDICINE?

Scientific method dictates that a new treatment must be fairly tested. Multiple experiments, repeated in more than one laboratory, must test and retest the treatment to determine its safety and effectiveness and to measure whether it works any better than a *placebo.*

The **placebo effect** predicts that *any* treatment will automatically make you feel better. For example, a sugar pill, a pain killer, and the doctor's hand touching your aching back are all likely to ease your pain. So when humans are involved, the experiment must be *double-blind*: neither the patient nor the experimenter must know what is being tested.

When the first data on CPAP were published by Sullivan's group in Australia in 1981,[1] the rest of the medical community was skeptical. Experiments were repeated in other labs around the world; the good results were verified. CPAP has now become a treatment principle that has shown results in many thousands of cases.

Now what about the "miracle of magnetism"? Let's run that notion through our rules of thumb. Does it seem too good to be true that tiny, weak magnetic fields could abolish the effects of sleep apnea? Does the "authority" selling this theory have medical credentials? Has he done double-blind experiments and published the results in a reputable medical journal? No. Who profits from the sale of the magnets? He does.

What do you think? Is there proof that magnets revitalized Mr. Chambers? Or was his improvement more likely the result of his new BiPAP™.

ALTERNATIVE MEDICINE: WHAT IT CAN AND CAN *NOT* DO

With a few exceptions, most alternative medical practices are not harmful, provided they are not used as a substitute for good primary medical care. They may be helpful in promoting better health. At worst, they may be needlessly costly. None can offer you the cure for sleep apnea.

If you feel compelled to try alternative methods, then at least be scientific about it: discuss your ideas with your doctor, do a controlled experiment yourself, and then be prepared to return to the sleep lab to find out whether there has been a measurable improvement in your sleep apnea.

TWO VERY BAD DECISIONS

One of the worst decisions you could make would be to stop using the treatment your sleep specialist prescribed while you try some new alternative.

If you want to experiment with unconventional treatments (provided they are not harmful), at least continue to use your CPAP at the same time.

If you stop using CPAP, your sleep apnea is guaranteed to return, and over time it will become worse.

The second bad decision would be to use an alternative practitioner as your primary or only doctor. Most alternative practitioners have limited medical training. They may fail to diagnose a serious disease (diabetes, cancer, heart condition) that could be fatal if it is not properly treated.

If you must experiment with alternatives, do so in addition to good, regular, conventional medical care.

BUT MAYBE *THIS* REALLY *IS* THE CURE!

It's true: the cure for sleep apnea may, indeed, exist in some obscure alternative medical treatment. Many scientific discoveries originate outside the conventional establishment.

The medical establishment is very slow to accept new ideas. Unconventional treatments are viewed with skepticism bordering on suspicion, and their proponents are often ostracized by the medical community.

Sleep disorders medicine itself is a perfect example of how long it takes to integrate a new concept into mainstream medicine. Sleep disorders research has been going on for more than 40 years, but today sleep disorders medicine is only beginning to be taught in medical schools.

Yet this very skepticism is what guards the public from the quacks. New medicine has to prove itself through scientific method and peer review in the medical journals. This process prevents abuse and exploitation of the public by incompetent scientists, unscrupulous industries, and personal greed.

The system isn't perfect. Some bad science is reported in the medical journals. Some good treatments take longer than they should to reach the patient. Progress seems slow; however, continual advances are being made. And examples of what can happen when the review process breaks down (e.g., thalido-mide) show us the value of deliberate skepticism and medical conservatism.

If a sure cure for sleep apnea exists today, the medical com-munity hasn't heard about it, much less had a chance to test it scientifically. Prudence suggests that we keep on using our CPAPs and remain patient and skeptical.

Summary

❖ *Rules of thumb for detecting medical quackery:*

> *Be skeptical.*
>
> *Ask for credentials.*
>
> *Know who profits and whether the product or service is worth the money.*
>
> *Learn whether the research followed scientific method.*

❖ *Keep using your CPAP, if you decide to try alternatives.*

❖ *Do not use an alternative practitioner as your only or primary physician.*

➤ ➤ ➤   APPENDIX   ➤ ➤ ➤

Addresses, Products, and Services for People with Sleep Apnea

The AWAKE Network

AWAKE is the national sleep apnea patient support network. Your sleep center's CPAP coordinator should know the nearest AWAKE group. If not, locate the nearest AWAKE group or obtain guidelines on starting an AWAKE group by contacting:

> AWAKE Network
> P.O. Box 66
> Belmont, MA 02178-0001

A nationwide list of AWAKE and other sleep apnea support groups on the Internet is being planned, as we go to press, by two Internet AWAKE home pages: New York and Chicago. (See "Sleep Apnea on the Internet," p. 209.) Other sleep disorders Web sites are expected to provide links to this list.

AMERICAN SLEEP APNEA ASSOCIATION (ASAA)

The American Sleep Apnea Association (ASAA) is a national membership organization for people with sleep apnea, dedicated to public education and support for medical advances in sleep apnea. Individual membership: $25. Quarterly newsletter. Contact via AWAKE Network address, above.

NATIONAL SLEEP FOUNDATION

This non-profit organization's mission is to improve the quality of life of people with sleep disorders and to prevent catastrophic accidents related to sleep deprivation and disorders.

The NSF publishes excellent brochures on each of the sleep disorders. For a copy of the sleep apnea brochure, send your request and a self-addressed, stamped, business-size envelope to:

National Sleep Foundation, Dept. SS
1367 Connecticut Avenue NW, Suite 200
Washington, D.C. 20036

AMERICAN SLEEP DISORDERS ASSOCIATION (ASDA)

The American Sleep Disorders Association (ASDA) is the professional sleep medicine organization, comprised of individual members and accredited member sleep centers and sleep laboratories. Contact them for a listing of accredited sleep centers.

American Sleep Disorders Association
1610 14th Street NW, Suite 300
Rochester, MN 55901–2200
507-287-6006

WAKE UP AMERICA

Wake Up America is a grassroots advocacy group that encourages citizen action in support of research and medical and public education on sleep disorders. To become involved, write:

Wake Up America
701 Welch Road, Suite 2226
Palo Alto, CA 94304

INTERNATIONAL SLEEP APNEA CONTACTS

Australia

Mr. Laurie Cree
Sleep Apnea Research Association (SARA)
73 Shirley Road
Roseville, NSW 2069, Australia
61 (2) 416-2372

Great Britain

Dr. C. D. Hanning
British Sleep Society
Sleep Disorder Clinic
Leicestershire General Hospital
Leicester, LE5 4PW
United Kingdom
0533-584-602

SLEEP APNEA ON THE INTERNET

Worldwide Web Pages (as of 9/95)

Sleep Medicine Homepage
  http://www.cloud9.net/~thorpy
Sleep Apnea Homepage
  http://www.access.digex.net/~faust/sldord
Sleepnet (Wake Up America, other resources, from Stanford
    School of Sleep Medicine)
  http://www.sleepnet.com

New York City AWAKE Home Page
http://www.bway.net/~marlene/awake.html

Message Boards

Prodigy
> Jump to Medical Support bulletin board under ... other
> Medical, subject...Sleep Apnea

America Online
> Clubs & Interests ... Better Health & Medicine ...
> Message Center ... General Health ... Sleep Apnea & zzz

Internet Sleep Disorders newsgroup
alt.support.sleep-disorders

JAW RETAINERS

Sleep Disorders Dental Society

For information about dentists in your region who are familiar with the use of oral appliances for treating sleep apnea, send your request and a stamped, self-addressed business envelope to:

Sleep Disorders Dental Society
11676 Perry Highway
Building 1, Suite 1204
Wexford, PA 15090

SLEEP POSITION

Monitor

For information about the effectiveness of changing sleep position as a treatment for sleep apnea and for information on sleep position monitors, check the following reference:

Cartwright, R. D. Effect of Sleep Position on Sleep Apnea Severity. *Sleep* 1984 7(2):110–114.

TRACHEOSTOMY

A Speaking Valve

A speaking valve can be attached to the outside of most trach tubes and is said to decrease the amount of mucous secretion that occurs with use of the standard tube. Apparently, the reason for this is that the one-way valve allows the wearer to exhale through the nose and mouth, which promotes the normal evaporation of moisture. The manufacturer does not recommend wearing the valve at night, but some patients have done so and report that it works fine and that they no longer have to worry about blowing out the trach tube several times a night. Check with your sleep specialist about this. For more information contact

Passy Muir Tracheostomy Speaking Valve
Passy-Muir, Inc.
4521 Campus Drive, Suite 273
Irvine, CA 92715
714-833-8255

Cleaning

For cleaning try Ivory Snow (no perfume), half-strength hydrogen peroxide, or a disinfectant/germicide called Control III, available from homecare companies (dilute as directed). Be sure to rinse well.

If you can't find a cleaning brush to fit inside your trach tube, the Kellog Brush Manufacturing Company (Easthampton, MA) makes a small brush for cleaning percolators that can be cut off and adapted.

If your tube is removable, the plastic containers for storing false teeth make good containers for washing and storing the tube.

Plugging and Sealing

For a plug try different types of earplugs of various sizes. One that fits some sizes of trach tube is Com-fit earplugs (Norton, Cerritus, CA).

For ties to secure the plate try Martin Trach-Secure (Diatek, San Diego) or a small elastic cord tied to a pair of hooks from a set of hooks-and-eyes.

For sealing the stoma during the day, try Stomahesive, made by Squibb for attaching colostomy bags, available in 4-inch squares from medical supply stores. Trim the squares to fit. If your skin is oily, try painting the area with benzoin before attaching the patch—this also makes the patch easier to remove. "Carry a spare patch in case of a blowout," warns one user.

WEIGHT LOSS

Good Sources of Sensible, Well-Balanced Recipes

The Pritikin Program for Diet and Exercise, by Nathan Pritikin with Patrick M. McGrady, Bantam. Excellent low-fat, low-sugar, low-salt, low-calorie, high-fiber recipes.

Don't Eat Your Heart Out Cookbook, by Joseph C. Piscatella, Workman Publishing. Good low-fat, low-salt, low-sugar recipes, not as low-calorie as Pritikin.

General Diet Guidelines

You can turn many of your favorite recipes into low-calorie recipes by doing the following:

1. Eliminate fats and oils (butter, margarine, other shortenings, dairy, and other animal fats). To keep food from sticking while cooking, use a nonstick pan. To sauté use a little water or bouillon instead of butter or oil. Refrigerate foods overnight and skim off the congealed fat the next day. Substitute low-fat or nonfat products for products high in fat: nonfat milk and

yogurt instead of regular; yogurt instead of sour cream; low-fat cheese such as part-skim mozzarella instead of fatty cheeses such as cheddar and jack; chicken or turkey instead of beef. Eat more seafood.

2. Cut down on sugar. Pritikin's recipes often use a small amount of frozen apple juice concentrate in place of sugar. This juice contains only a small amount of sugar and adds just the right hint of sweetness.

3. Cut down on salt. Use herbs instead.

4. Eat lots of fresh vegetables and fruits. They are bulky and fill you up, they are low in calories, and they are full of vitamins and minerals.

5. Use whole-grain products (flour, bread, rice, pasta, and so on) instead of highly refined products. Whole-grain products are bulkier, so you will feel full on fewer calories.

You can actually have fun inventing your own low-calorie versions of favorite recipes, using more healthful substitutions. Exercising your creativity in the kitchen makes dieting more enjoyable. You can design your own great weight loss recipes.

DRUGS THAT CAN MAKE SLEEP APNEA WORSE

Many medications can make sleep apnea worse by making you drowsy or by disturbing your sleep or breathing. Discuss all your medications with your sleep specialist. He may want to adjust dosages or suggest alternatives.

Some common *over-the-counter (nonprescription)* drugs, such as antihistamines, can make sleep apnea worse. Ask your pharmacist about all nonprescription medications that you take frequently. Can they cause drowsiness, breathing problems, or insomnia? Can he suggest alternative medications with fewer side effects?

The following *prescription* drugs can cause problems for people with sleep apnea. If you are taking any of these (or the generic form of the same drug), be sure to discuss them with your sleep physician.

TABLE: *Drugs That Can Cause DROWSINESS or APNEA or INSOMNIA*

The **xs** indicate the chances that a person taking the drug will experience
the problem listed. (Based on data from *Physicians Desk Reference*, 1993.)
x = small chance (problem affects fewer than 10% of people taking the
drug)
xx = moderate chance (problem affects 10% to 25% of people taking the
drug)
xxx = common problem (affects more than 25% of people taking the drug)

	DROWSINESS	APNEA	INSOMNIA
Actifed with Codeine Cough Syr.	xxx		
Alfenta		x	
Alferon N	xx		
Ambien	xx		
Anafranil	xxx		xx
Anaprox, Anaprox DS	x		
Anestacon	xxx		
Asendin	xx		
Atgam		xx	
Atrofen	xxx		x
Benadryl	xxx		xxx
Bentyl	x		
Buspar	xx		x
Cardura	x		
Catapres, Catapres TTS	xxx		
Centrax	x		
CHEMET	xx		
Clozaril	xxx		
Combipres	xxx		
Cylert			xxx
Cytadren	xxx		
DHC Plus	xxx		
Dantrium	xxx		

	DROWSINESS	APNEA	INSOMNIA
Depo-Provera			x
Desyrel	xxx		x
Dilantin with Phenobarbital	xxx		
Doral	xx		
Duragesic	xx	xx	
Emcyt			x
Emete-con	xxx		
Empirin with Codeine	xxx		
Ergamisol	x		
Esgic-Plus	xxx		
Exosurf		xxx	
Fioricet	xxx		
Fiorinal	xxx		
Flexeril	xxx		
Floxin			x
Habitrol	x		x
Halcion	xx		
Hismanal	x		
Hylorel	xx		
Hytrin	x		
IFEX	xxx		
Innovar		xxx	
Intron A	x		x
Kerlone			x
Klonopin	xxx		
Limbitrol, Limbitrol DS	xxx		
Lioresal	xxx		x
Lopressor HCT	xx		
Ludiomil	xx		
Lupron			x
Lysodren	xxx		

	DROWSINESS	APNEA	INSOMNIA
Marinol (Dronabinol)	xx		
Marplan			xxx
Mazicon			x
Mepron			xx
Minipress	x		
Minizide	x		
Moban	xxx		
Nalfon 200	x		
Naprosyn	x		
Nicoderm			xx
Orudis			x
Parlodel	x		
Paxil	xx		xx
PedvaxHIB	xxx		
Permax	xx		x
Phenurone	x		
Phrenilin	xxx		
ProSom	xxx		
Prostep	x		x
Prostin VR		xx	
Prozac	xx		xx
Pyridium Plus	xxx		
Reglan	xx		
Restoril	xx		
Retrovir	x		x
Ritalin			xxx
Rynatan, Rynatan-S	xxx		
Rynatuss	xxx		
Sanorex			xxx
Seconal	xxx		
Sectral			x
Sedapap	xxx		

	DROWSINESS	APNEA	INSOMNIA
Seldane, Seldane-D	x		xxx
Sinequan	xxx		
Soma, Soma with Codeine	xxx		
Stadol	xxx		xx
Suprane		xx	
Survanta		xxx	
Symmetrel			xx
Synarel			x
Tavist, Tavist-1, Tavist-D	xxx		
Tegretol	xxx		
Temaril	xxx		
Tenex	xxx		x
Theo-X			xxx
Toradol	x		xx
Trandate	x		
Transderm Scop	x		
Tranxene, Tranxene-SD	xxx		
Trinalin	xxx		
Tripedia	xx		
Valrelease	xxx		
Ventolin			x
Versed		xx	
Videx			xxx
Visken			xx
Wellbutrin			xx
Wytensin	xx		
Xanax	xxx		xxx
Xylocaine	xxx		
Zoladex			x
Zoloft	xx		xx

REFERENCES

CHAPTER 1

1. Young, Terry, Mari Palta, Jerome Dempsey, James Skatrud, Steven Weber, and Safwan Badr. The occurrence of sleep-disordered breathing among middle-paged adults. *N Engl J Med* 1993;328(17):1230–1235.
2. Dement, William. *Statement on the Findings and Recommendations of the National Commission on Sleep Disorders Research*, Field hearing before U.S. Senate Appropriations Committee, Portland, OR, November 4, 1992.

CHAPTER 2

1. Aldrich, Michael S. Automobile accidents in patients with sleep disorders. *Sleep* 1989;12(6):487–494.
2. Stoohs, R., L. Bingham, A. Itoi, C. Guilleminault, and W. C. Dement. Cross-sectional study of the prevalence of OSA in a population of long-haul truck drivers. Reported at the European Sleep Research Society meeting in Helsinki, 1992.
3. Watson, Robert, Glen Greenberg, Dennis Deptula. Neurophysiological deficits in sleep apnea (abstract). In *Sleep Research*, Vol. 14, p. 136. Edited by Michael Chase. Los Angeles: UCLA Brain Information Service/Brain Research Institute, 1985.
4. Fairbanks, David. Snoring: an overview. In *Snoring and Obstructive Sleep Apnea*. Edited by David Fairbanks, Shiro Fujita, T. Ikematsu, and F. B. Simmons. New York: Raven, 1987.
5. Shepard, John W. Pathophysiology and medical therapy of sleep apnea. *Ear Nose Throat J* 1984 May 63(5):198–212.
6. Strohl, Kingman P., Colin E. Sullivan, and Nicholas A. Saunders. Sleep apnea syndromes. In *Sleep and Breathing*. Edited by Nicholas A. Saunders and Colin E. Sullivan. Lung Biology in Health and Disease Series, Vol. 21. New York: Marcel Dekker, 1984.
7. Harper, Ronald M. Obstructive sleep apnea. In *Hypoxia, Exercise, and Altitude:* Proceedings of the 3rd International Hypoxia Symposium, pp. 97–105. Progress in Clinical and Biological Research Series, Vol. 136. New York: Liss, 1983.

8. Guilleminault, Christian, and William C. Dement. Sleep apnea syndromes and related sleep disorders. In *Sleep Disorders: Diagnosis and Treatment.* Edited by Robert L. Williams and Ismet Karacan. New York: Wiley, 1978.
9. Kohler U., J. Mayer, J. H. Peter, and P. v. Wichert. Cardiac arrhythmias accompanying sleep apnea activity (SAA) in patients with established sleep apnea and in general outpatients (abstract). In *Sleep Research*, Vol. 14, p. 179. Edited by Michael Chase. Los Angeles: UCLA Brain Information Service/Brain Research Institute, 1985.
10. Jennum, Poul, Kirsten Schultz-Larsen, and Gordon Wildscheidtz. Snoring as a medical risk factor. IV. Relation to lung function and hemoglobin concentration (abstract). In *Sleep Research*, Vol. 14, p. 173. Edited by Michael Chase. Los Angeles: UCLA Brain Information Service/Brain Research Institute, 1985.
11. Podszus, Th., J. Mayer, Th. Penzel, J.H. Peter, P. v. Wichert. Hemodynamics during sleep in patients with sleep apnea (abstract). In Sleep Research, Vol. 14, p. 198. Edited by Michael Chase. Los Angeles: UCLA Brain Information Service/Brain Research Institute, 1985.
12. Cartwright, Rosalind, and Sara Knight. Silent partners: the wives of sleep apneic patients. *Sleep* 1987;10(3):244–248.
13. Guilleminault, Christian, and Elio Lugaresi. *Sleep/Wake Disorders: Natural History, Epidemiology, and Long-Term Evolution.* New York: Raven, 1983.
14. Lavie, Peretz, and A.E. Rubin. Effects of nasal occlusion on respiration in sleep: evidence of inheritability of sleep apnea proneness. *Acta Otolaryngol* (Stockh) 1984 Jan-Feb;97(1–2):127–130.
15. Young, Terry, Mari Palta, Jerome Dempsey, James Skatrud, Steven Weber, and Safwan Badr. The occurrence of sleep-disordered breathing among middle-aged adults. *N Engl J Med* 1993;328(17):1230–1235.
16. Dement, William C. *Some Must Watch While Some Must Sleep.* San Francisco: W.H. Freeman, 1972.
17. Orr, William C. Utilization of polysomnography in the assessment of sleep disorders. *Med Clin North Am* 1985;69(6):1153–1167.
18. Lavie, Peretz. Sleep apnea in industrial workers. In *Sleep/Wake Disorders: Natural History, Epidemiology, and Long-Term Evolution.* New York: Raven, 1983.
19. Hales, Dianne. *The Complete Book of Sleep: How Your Nights Affect Your Days* Reading, Mass.: Addison–Wesley, 1981.

CHAPTER 3

1. Dement, William C. *Some Must Watch While Some Must Sleep.* San Francisco: W.H. Freeman, 1972.
2. Shepard, John W. Pathophysiology and medical therapy of sleep apnea. *Ear Nose Throat J* 1984 May 63(5):198–212.
3. Lugaresi, E., S. Mondini, M. Zucconi, P. Montagna, F. Cirignotta. Staging of heavy snorers' disease: a proposal. In Proceedings of the 4th International Congress of Sleep Research Satellite Symposium (Bologna). *Bull Eur Physiopathol Respir* 1983;19(6):590–594.

CHAPTER 4

1. Guilleminault, Christian, M.D.. Stanford Sleep Disorders Center, Stanford. California. Interview, 28 March 1986.
2. Jamieson, Andrew. C. Guilleminault, M. Partinen, and M. A. Quera–Salva. Obstructive sleep apnea patients have craniomandibular abnormalities. *Sleep* 1986;9(4):469–477.
3. Shepard, John W. Pathophysiology and medical therapy of sleep apnea. *Ear Nose Throat J* 1984 May 63(5):198–212.

CHAPTER 5

1. Dement, William. *Statement on the Findings and Recommendations of the National Commission on Sleep Disorders Research*, Field hearing before U.S. Senate Appropriations Committee, Portland, OR, November 4, 1992.

CHAPTER 7

1. Colman M. F. Limitations, pitfalls, and risk management in palatopharyngoplasty. In *Snoring and Obstructive Sleep Apnea*. Edited by David Fairbanks, Shiro Fujita, T. Ikematsu, and F.B. Simmons. New York: Raven, 1987.
2. Thawley, Stanley E. Surgical treatment of obstructive sleep apnea. *Med Clin North Am* 1985;69(6):1337–1357.
3. White, David P., Clifford W. Zwillich, Cheryl K. Pickett, Neil J. Douglas, Larry J. Findley, and John V. Weil. Central sleep apnea: improvement with acetazolamide therapy. *Arch Intern Med* 1982 Oct;142:1816–1819.
4. Whyte, K. F., G. A. Gould, M. A. A. Airlie, C. M. Shapiro, and N. J. Douglas. Role of protriptyline and acetazolamide in sleep apnea/hypopnea syndrome. *Sleep* 1988;11(5):463–472.
5. Shore, Eric T., and Richard P. Millman. Central sleep apnea and acetazolamide therapy (letter). *Arch Intern Med* 1983 June;143:1278, 1280.
6. Guilleminault, Christian, and William C. Dement. Sleep apnea syndromes and related sleep disorders. In *Sleep Disorders: Diagnosis and Treatment*. Edited by Robert L. Williams and Ismet Karacan. New York: Wiley, 1978.
7. Guilleminault, Christian, Johanna van den Hoed, and Merrill M. Mitler. Clinical overview of the sleep apnea syndromes. In *Sleep Apnea Syndromes*, Kroc Foundation Series, Vol. 11. Edited by Christian Guilleminault and William C. Dement. New York: Liss, 1978.
8. Gotfried, Mark H., and Stuart F. Quan. Obstructive sleep apnea - pathogenesis and treatment. *Lung* 1984;162:1–13.
9. Schmidt, H. L–Tryptophan in the treatment of impaired respiration in sleep. In Proceedings of the 4th International Congress of Sleep Research Satellite Symposium (Bologna). *Bull Eur Physiopathol Respir* 1983;19(6):625–629.

10. Krieger, J., P. Mangin, and D. Kurtz. Effects of almitrine in the treatment of sleep apnea syndromes. In Proceedings of the 4th International Congress of Sleep Research Satellite Symposium (Bologna). *Bull Eur Physiopathol Respir* 1983;19(6):630.

11. Douglas, N. J., J. J. Connaughton, A. D. Morgan, C. N. Shapiro, N. Pauly, and D.C. Flenly. Effect of almitrine on nocturnal hypoxaemia in chronic bronchitis and emphysema, and in patients with central sleep apnea. In Proceedings of the 4th International Congress of Sleep Research Satellite Symposium (Bologna). *Bull Eur Physiopathol Respir* 1983;19(6):631.

12. Krieger, J., P. Mangin, and D. Kurtz. Almitrine and sleep apnea. *Lancet* 1982 July 24;9(8291):210.

13. White, David P. Central sleep apnea. *Med Clin North Am* 1985;69(6): 1205–1219.

14. Meisner H., J. G. Schober, E. Struck, B. Lipowski, P. Mayser, and F. Sebening. Phrenic nerve pacing for the treatment of central hypoventilation syndrome—state of the art and case report. *Thorac Cardiovasc Surgeon* 1983;31:21–25.

15. Brouillette, Robert T., Michel N. Ilbawi, and Carl E. Hunt. Phrenic nerve pacing in infants and children: a review of experience and report on the usefulness of phrenic nerve stimulation studies. *J Pediatrics* 1983 Jan;102(1):32–39.

16. Glenn, William W. L., Mildred Phelps, and Larry M. Gersten. Diaphragm pacing in the management of central alveolar hypoventilation. In *Sleep Apnea Syndromes*, Kroc Foundation Series, Vol. 11. Edited by Christian Guilleminault and William C. Dement. New York: Liss, 1978.

17. Sullivan, Colin E., Michael Berthon–Jones, Faiq G. Issa, and Lorraine Eves. Reversal of obstructive sleep apnoea by continuous positive airway pressure applied through the nares. *Lancet* 1981 April 18;1(8225):862–865.

18. Issa, Faiq G, and Colin E. Sullivan. Reversal of central apnea using nasal CPAP. *Chest* 1986;90(2):165–176.

19. Burwell C. Sidney, Eugene D. Robin, Robert D. Whaley, and Albert G. Bikelman. Extreme obesity associated with alveolar hypoventilation - a Pickwickian syndrome. *Am J Med* 1956;21:811–818.

20. Jung, Richard, and Wolfgang Kuhlo. Neurophysiological studies of abnormal night sleep in the Pickwickian syndrome. *Progress in Brain Research: Sleep Mechanisms* 1965;18:140–159.

21. Rinke, Carlotta. Shedding a little light on sleep disorders. *JAMA* 1981 Feb;245(6):549.

22. Sanders, Mark H., Cynthia A. Gruendl, and Robert M. Rogers. Patient compliance with nasal CPAP therapy for sleep apnea. *Chest* 1986;90(3):330–333.

23. Cartwright, R. D., and C. F. Samelson. Effects of a non-surgical treatment for obstructive sleep apnea - the tongue-retaining device. *JAMA* 1982;248(6):705–709.

24. Cartwright, Rosalind D. Predicting response to the tongue retaining device for sleep apnea syndrome. *Arch Otolaryngol* 1985;111:385–388.

25. Soll, Bruce A., and Peter T. George. Treatment of obstructive sleep apnea with a nocturnal airway-patency appliance. *New Engl J Med.* 1985;313(6):386, 387.

26. Andrews, J. N., Christian Guilleminault, and R. A. Holdaway. Retaining devices and mandibular positioning appliances. In Proceedings of the 4th International Congress of Sleep Research Satellite Symposium (Bologna). *Bull Eur Physiopathol Respir* 1983;19(6):611.

27. American Sleep Disorders Association. Standards of Practice Committee. Practice parameters for the treatment of snoring and obstructive sleep apnea with oral appliances. *Sleep* 1995;18(6):511–513.

28. Brownell, L. G., R. Perez-Padilla, P. West, and M. H. Kryger. The role of protriptyline in obstructive sleep apnea. In Proceedings of the 4th International Congress of Sleep Research Satellite Symposium (Bologna). *Bull Eur Physiopathol Respir* 1983;19(6):621–624.

29. Guilleminault, C., and S. Mondini. Need for multi-diagnostic approaches before considering treatment in obstructive sleep apnea. In Proceedings of the 4th International Congress of Sleep Research Satellite Symposium (Bologna). *Bull Eur Physiopathol Respir* 1983;19(6):583–589.

30. Smith, Philip L., Edward F. Haponik, Richard P. Allen, and Eugene R. Bleecker. The effects of protriptyline in sleep-disordered breathing. *Am Rev Respir Dis* 1983;127:8–13.

31. Conway, W., S. Fujita, F. Zorick, K. Sicklesteel, T. Roehrs, R. Wittig, and T. Roth. Uvulopalatopharyngoplasty: one-year follow-up. *Chest* 1985 Sept; 88(3):385–387.

32. Guilleminault, C., B. Hayes, L. Smith, and F. B. Simmons. Palatopharyngoplasty and obstructive sleep apnea syndrome. In Proceedings of the 4th International Congress of Sleep Research Satellite Symposium (Bologna). *Bull Eur Physiopathol Respir* 1983;19(6):595–599.

33. Katsantonis, George P., James K. Walsh, Paula K. Schweitzer, and William H. Friedman. Further evaluation of uvulopalatopharyngoplasty in the treatment of obstructive sleep apnea syndrome. *Otolaryngol Head Neck Surg* 1985 April;93(2):244–250.

34. Fujita, Shiro, William A. Conway, Frank J. Zorick, Jeanne M. Sicklesteel, Timothy A. Roehrs, Robert M. Wittig, and Thomas Roth. Evaluation of the effectiveness of uvulopalatopharyngoplasty. *Laryngoscope* 1985 Jan;95:70–74.

35. Riley, R., C. Guilleminault, N. Powell, and F. Blair Simmons. Palatopharyngoplasty failure, cephalometric roentgenograms, and obstructive sleep apnea. *Otolaryngol Head Neck Surg* 1985 April;93(2):240–243.

36. Riley, Robert, Christian Guilleminault, Juan Herran, and Nelson Powell. Cephalometric analyses and flow-volume loops in obstructive sleep apnea patients. *Sleep* 1983;6(4):303–311.

37. Jamieson, Andrew, C. Guilleminault, M. Partinen, and M. A. Quera–Salva. Obstructive sleep apnea patients have craniomandibular abnormalities. *Sleep* 1986;9(4):469–477.

38. Moran, W. B., Jr. Obstructive sleep apnea: diagnosis by history, physical exam, and special studies. In *Snoring and Obstructive Sleep Apnea.* Edited by David Fairbanks, Shiro Fujita, T. Ikematsu, and F. B. Simmons. New York: Raven, 1987.

39. Shepard, John W., Jr., Warren B. Gefter, Christian Guilleminault, Eric A. Hoffman, Victor Hoffstein, David W. Hudgel, Paul M. Suratt, and David P. White. Evaluation of the upper airway in patients with obstructive sleep apnea. *Sleep* 1991;14(4):361–371.

40. Riley, R., C. Guilleminault, N. Powell, and S. Derman. Mandibular osteotomy and hyoid bone advancement for obstructive sleep apnea: a case report. *Sleep* 1984;7(1):79–82.

41. Powell, N., C. Guilleminault, R. Riley, and L. Smith. Mandibular advancement and obstructive sleep apnea synbdrome. In Proceedings of the 4th International Congress of Sleep Research Satellite Symposium (Bologna). *Bull Eur Physiopathol Respir* 1983;19(6):607–610.

42. Guilleminault, Christian, F. Blair Simmons, Jorge Motta, Joseph Cummiskey, Mark Rosekind, John S. Schroeder, and William C. Dement. Obstructive sleep apnea syndrome and tracheostomy: long-term follow-up experience. *Arch Intern Med* 1981;141:985–988.

43. Dye, John P., and L. Jack Faling. Living with a tracheostomy for sleep apnea (letters). *N Engl J Med* 1983 May;308(19):1167, 1168.

44. Lubin, M. F., H. K. Walker, and R. B. Smith, III, eds. *Medical Management of the Surgical Patient.* 2nd ed. London: Butterworths, 1988.

45. Charuzi, Ilan, Amnon Ovnat, Jochanan Peiser, Hedy Saltz, Simon Weitzman, and Peretz Lavie. The effect of surgical weight reduction on sleep quality in obesity-related sleep apnea syndrome. *Surgery* 1985 May;97(5):535–538.

46. Penek, J. Laser-assisted uvulopalatoplasty: the cart before the horse. *Chest* 1995;107(1):1–3.

47. American Sleep Disorders Association. Standards of Practice Committee. Practice parameters for the use of laser-assisted uvulopalatoplasty. *Sleep* 1994;17(8):744–748.

CHAPTER 8

1. Waldhorn, R.E. Cardiopulmonary consequences of obstructive sleep apnea. In *Snoring and Obstructive Sleep Apnea.* Edited by David Fairbanks, Shiro Fujita, T. Ikematsu, and F.B. Simmons. New York: Raven, 1987.

2. Kryger, Meir H. Sleep apnea: from the needles of Dionysius to continuous positive airway pressure. *Arch Intern Med* 1983 Dec;143(12):2301–2303.

3. Lavie, Peretz. Nothing new under the moon: historical accounts of sleep apnea syndrome. *Arch Intern Med* 1984 Oct;144(10):2025–2028.

4. Gastaut, H., C. A. Tassinari, and B. Duron. Polygraphic study of the episodic diurnal and nocturnal (hypnic and respiratory) manifestations of the Pickwick syndrome. *Brain Research* 1966;2:167–186.

5. Jung, Richard, and Wolfgang Kuhlo. Neurophysiological studies of abnormal night sleep in the Pickwickian syndrome. *Progress in Brain Research: Sleep Mechanisms* 1965;18:140–159.
6. Charuzi, Ilan, Amnon Ovnat, Jochanan Peiser, Hedy Saltz, Simon Weitzman, and Peretz Lavie. The effect of surgical weight reduction on sleep quality in obesity-related sleep apnea syndrome. *Surgery* 1985 May;97(5):535–538.
7. Burwell C. Sidney, Eugene D. Robin, Robert D. Whaley, and Albert G. Bikelman. Extreme obesity associated with alveolar hypoventilation—a Pickwickian syndrome. *Am J Med* 1956;21:811–818.
8. Sullivan, Colin E., M. Berthon-Jones, and F. G. Issa. Remission of severe obesity-hypoventilation syndrome after short-term treatment during sleep with nasal continuous positive airway pressure. *Am Rev Respir Dis* 1983 July;128(1):177–181.

CHAPTER 9

1. Sullivan, Colin E. Personal Communication. 1993. His belief in the link between SIDS and OSA is based on his own recent experience and data from Kahn's group in Belgium.
2. Limerick, The Countess of. Greetings. In *Sudden Infant Death Syndrome:* Proceedings of the 1982 International Research Conference (Baltimore). Edited by J. Tyson Tildon, Lois M. Roeder, and Alfred Steinschneider. New York: Academic, 1983.
3. Hodgman, Joan E., and Toke Hoppenbrouwers. Cardiorespiratory behavior in infants at increased epidemiological risk for SIDS. In *Sudden Infant Death Syndrome*: Proceedings of the 1982 International Research Conference (Baltimore). Edited by J. Tyson Tildon, Lois M. Roeder, and Alfred Steinschneider. New York: Academic, 1983.
4. Albani, M., K. H. P. Bentele, C. Budde, and F. J. Schulte. Infant sleep apnea profile: preterm vs. term infants. *Eur J Pediatrics* 1985 March; 143(4):261–268.
5. Guilleminault, Christian. Sleep apnea in the full-term infant. In *Sleep and Its Disorders in Children.* Edited by Christian Guilleminault. New York: Raven, 1987.
6. Golding, Jean, Sylvia Limerick, and Aidan Macfarlane. *Sudden Infant Death: Patterns, Puzzles, and Problems.* Seattle: University of Washington Press, 1985.

CHAPTER 10

1. Ferber, Richard, M.D. *Solve Your Child's Sleep Problems.* New York: Simon and Schuster, 1985.
2. Guilleminault, Christian. Obstructive sleep apnea syndrome in children. In *Sleep and Its Disorders in Children.* Edited by Christian Guilleminault. New York: Raven, 1987.

3. Guilleminault, Christian, and Ronald Ariagno. Apnea during sleep in infants and children. In *Principles and Practice of Sleep Medicine*, Meir H. Kryger, Thomas Roth, and William C. Dement. Philadelphia: W.B.Saunders, 1989.

CHAPTER 11

1. Prinz, Patricia N., and Murray Raskind. Aging and sleep disorders. In *Sleep Disorders: Diagnosis and Treatment.* Edited by Robert L. Williams and Ismet Karacan. New York: Wiley, 1978.
2. Ancoli-Israel, Sonia, Daniel F. Kriicpke, William Mason, and Oscar J. Kaplan. Sleep apnea and periodic movements in an aging sample. *J Gerontol* 1985;40(4):419–425.
3. Carskadon, Mary A., and William C. Dement. Respiration during sleep in the aged human. *J Gerontol* 1981;36(4):420–423.
4. Bliwise, Donald L., and Ralph A. Pascualy. Sleep-related respiratory disturbance in elderly persons. *Compr Ther* 1984;10(7):8–14.

CHAPTER 14

1. Norman, Susan E., and Martin A. Cohn. Follow-up care at sleep disorders centers: a commitment beyond diagnosis (letter). *Sleep* 1985;8(1):71–73.

CHAPTER 16

1. Sullivan, Colin E., Michael Berthon-Jones, Faiq G. Issa, and Lorraine Eves. Reversal of obstructive sleep apnoea by continuous positive airway pressure applied through the nares. *Lancet* 1981 April 18;1(8225):862–865.

GLOSSARY

adenoids Similar to tonsils, but located behind and above the tonsils.

airway The passage through which air travels as it moves to and from your lungs. Your airway includes nose and mouth, throat, and the bronchial tubes that lead to your lungs.

angina pectoris Chest pain that occurs when the heart muscle does not get enough oxygen.

apnea Failure to move air in and out of your airway.

apnea event A failure to breathe that lasts for more than 10 seconds.

apnea index The number of apnea events per hour. A measure of the severity of sleep apnea.

apnea-plus-hypopnea index The total number of apnea and hypopnea events per hour. A measure of the severity of sleep apnea.

arrhythmia Variation from the normal rhythm of the heartbeat.

breathing center A center in your brain that controls the speed and forcefulness of your breathing.

CPAP Continuous positive airway pressure. A breathing system used to treat obstructive sleep apnea and other respiratory disorders.

carbon dioxide The waste gas produced by your body. It is removed from your blood stream in the lungs and leaves the body when you exhale.

cardiovascular Having to do with the heart or circulatory system.

carotid body A sensory structure in the carotid artery in the neck that measures the amount of oxygen in your blood and sends signals to the breathing center in your brain.

central sleep apnea   Sleep apnea that is caused by some irregularity in the brain's control of breathing.

cephalometry   Measurement of the size and location of the structures in the head, using x-rays or other imaging systems.

cuirass   A breathing device that fits over a patient's chest and helps him breathe. Sometimes used to treat central sleep apnea.

deviated septum   An irregularly shaped nasal septum, which may partly block the passage of air and interfere with breathing. *See* nasal septum.

diaphragm   The muscular wall that separates the chest cavity from the abdominal cavity. Your diaphragm is part of your breathing system; the downward contraction of the diaphragm muscles allows your lungs to expand and fill with air.

EDS   Excessive daytime sleepiness.

ENT specialist   Ear, nose, and throat specialist. Also called an otolaryngologist.

gastric bypass   A surgical procedure in which the stomach is stapled to make it smaller. Used to promote weight loss in morbidly obese patients.

hypertension   High blood pressure.

hypopnea   Shallow breathing in which the airflow in and out of the airway is less than half of normal.

larynx   The "voice box"; the structure in the lower throat that contains the vocal cords. The Adam's apple is the front of your larynx.

LAUP   Laser assisted uvulopalatoplasty. Laser surgery performed on the soft palate to reduce snoring. Not recommended for sleep apnea.

mandible   Lower jawbone.

mandibular reconstruction   Surgery to reshape the lower jaw.

maxilla   Upper jawbone.

maxillofacial surgery   Surgery on the upper jaw and face.

medulla, or medulla oblongata. A deep, primitive part of the brain. Sensors that detect carbon dioxide are located here. These sensors are involved in your breathing reflex.

mixed sleep apnea   Sleep apnea that is a combination of obstructive and central apnea.

nREM sleep Non-REM sleep. *See* REM sleep.

nasal septum The divider between the right and left nose cavities. It is made up of bone, cartilage, and soft tissue.

neurologic Having to do with the nervous system.

nocturnal Occurring at night.

obese Having a weight of more than 20% above the ideal body weight.

obstructive sleep apnea Sleep apnea caused by a blockage of the airway.

otolaryngologist An ear, nose, and throat specialist; also called an ENT specialist.

oxygen A gas that makes up 20% of the air your breathe. It is picked up in your lungs by red blood cells and carried throughout your body. All your body's cells need oxygen in order to live.

oxygen saturation The amount of oxygen being carried in your blood. Often used as a measure of the severity of sleep apnea. Normal oxygen saturation is about 95%, with some decrease with age.

pharynx The part of the throat just behind the mouth.

polycythemia An abnormal excess of red blood cells.

polysomnography The recording of a person's breathing, heartbeat, brain activity, body movements, and other physiologic signs during sleep.

pulmonary Having to do with the lungs.

RDI Respiratory Disturbance Index. A measure of the severity of sleep apnea. Equal to the number of apneas plus hypopneas, divided by total sleep time, and multiplied by 60.

red blood cells The cells that carry oxygen through the blood stream.

REM sleep The "rapid eye movement" stage of sleep. The "active" stage of sleep, during which the most vivid dreams occur.

set point The amount of carbon dioxide or oxygen in your blood that triggers the breathing center to make you inhale.

sleep apnea A condition in which a person stops breathing while asleep.

sleep latency The amount of time it takes for you to fall asleep. Indicates the degree of excessive daytime sleepiness.

soft palate   The flexible back part of the roof of your mouth.

tonsils   A pair of small glands located at the back of the mouth, on either side of the opening into the throat.

UPPP   Uvulopalatopharyngoplasty. A type of surgery sometimes used to treat snoring and obstructive sleep apnea.

uvula   The dangly, tongue-shaped tab that hangs down from the soft palate, at the back of your mouth.

Subject Index